Blunt Abdominal Trauma in Children

Rizwan Ahmad Khan • Shagufta Wahab
Editors

Blunt Abdominal Trauma in Children

Problems and Solutions

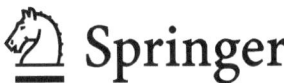 Springer

Editors
Rizwan Ahmad Khan
Department of Pediatric Surgery
Jawaharlal Nehru Medical College
Aligarh Muslim University
Aligarh
Uttar Pradesh
India

Shagufta Wahab
Department of Radio-diagnosis
Jawaharlal Nehru Medical College
Aligarh Muslim University
Aligarh
Uttar Pradesh
India

ISBN 978-981-13-0691-4   ISBN 978-981-13-0692-1   (eBook)
https://doi.org/10.1007/978-981-13-0692-1

Library of Congress Control Number: 2018945866

Printed on acid-free paper

This Springer imprint is published by the registered company Springer Nature Singapore Pte Ltd.
The registered company address is: 152 Beach Road, #21-01/04 Gateway East, Singapore 189721, Singapore

Foreword

As a pediatric surgeon involved with medical teaching in one of the most premier medical institutes of India, it cannot be more gratifying for me to learn that one of my bright students is bringing out a detailed in-depth book on pediatric abdominal trauma—one of the most frequently encountered scenarios in a casualty and also one of the most challenging.

My association with Dr. Rizwan goes back to 2005 when he joined our institute as an M.Ch student and impressed us with his dedication and hard work. It was during one of our casual discussions about 2 years ago that he and Dr. Shagufta felt about the lack of a detailed research publication on pediatric trauma. Most of the available publications have scratched the topic superficially only and detailed analysis of the demographics, etiology, prevention, initial presentation, clinical evaluation, imaging, management, and finally psychological post-trauma management has been lacking. They shared their experience with their colleagues in other medical institutes and finally came out with this wonderful book on pediatric abdominal trauma after 2 years of painstaking work, and I was really impressed with the extensiveness of the draft. As many medical authors realize, producing a book is a patient, tiresome, and lonely experience and many a times wonderful projects are lost along the way. But this project saw the light of day by the Grace of the Almighty and the efforts of the authors and editors—conceptualizing, drafting, redrafting, revising… the list is long. I congratulate them all for this wonderful work on pediatric abdominal trauma, which I hope will be of great help to all medical professionals and will guide better and complete patient management.

After more than a decade, it has been a wonderful experience to get associated with your former student and I am indeed honored to write the foreword for this book and wish it all the success.

Ram Samujh
Department of Pediatric Surgery
Advanced Pediatric Centre, Postgraduate Institute of Medical Education
and Research (PGIMER)
Chandigarh, India

Preface

Trauma constitutes a major part of everyday emergency that surgeons face all over the world. In today's world, where violence, intentional or unintentional, is increasingly getting common and prevalent, children being the vulnerable populace are becoming the innocent victims in alarmingly large numbers.

Penetrating trauma being easily identifiable is quickly diagnosed and also identified by nonmedical personnel as well as the general population and compels urgent and adequate measures. The blunt trauma to abdomen is not overtly visible and therefore gives a false impression to nonprofessionals as well as the general population that the child has "escaped unhurt." It also tests the clinical acumen of the best pediatric surgeons and radiologists as well.

When we decided to write on the diagnosis and management of blunt trauma abdomen in children, we realized that the topic, although niche, is quite exhaustive. However, such a book dealing with epidemiological aspects, risk factors, clinical and imaging aspect of injuries, their complications, and management could fulfill the existing gaps and provide a comprehensive knowledge on management aspects of blunt abdominal trauma in children.

In children, blunt nature of injuries is much more common than penetrating type. And 5–10% of children affected with blunt abdominal trauma sustain some form of intra-abdominal injury. Even among pediatric age groups (infants vs. school-aged children), there may be different mechanisms and presentation. Therefore, the problems and strategies of blunt trauma in adults cannot be extrapolated to pediatric age group because of variable anatomical, physiological, mechanical, and clinical aspects.

In fact, there are disparities based on socioeconomic and ethnic aspects also. Thus, clinical approach to a child with blunt abdominal trauma is nothing short of opening a Pandora's Box. It requires specialized and standardized methodology so as to give the best possible trauma care to the children.

With these points in mind, we undertook the task of bringing out this multi-authored book by the experts in their fields. The book consists of 14 chapters beginning with introduction and epidemiology of pediatric abdominal trauma, various steps in accurate diagnosis, management both surgical and nonsurgical, complication, and sequelae of the management. Finally, we also included a full-length chapter on psychological rehabilitation of these trauma patients and their families. The best aspect of this book is that we have tried to amalgamate the old knowledge and wisdom with updated and latest developments in the field of study because of which there might be some repetitions along the text. We have incorporated an elaborate bibliography to assist the reader for further reading and reference.

Our book not only covers pediatric blunt abdominal trauma and its management but also covers issues concerning trauma prevention and the post-trauma psychological issues in children and their families. It provides a comprehensive and holistic approach very much needed in pediatric care.

The editors wish that this book be useful for clinicians, radiologists, pediatricians, primary caregivers, pediatric surgeons, trauma trainees, and surgical as well as pediatric surgical residents and pediatric clinical psychologists.

In the end, we would like to acknowledge the efforts of Springer Nature and Springer personnel for their expert advice and guidance in producing this book.

We thank families of our contributors and our family for their unstinted support and patience. Last but not least, we feel gratitude for our "young patients" who were the cornerstone of this idea during the course of their care and hospital stay, and we sincerely hope and wish that our book will be helpful in improving the care of these very children.

Aligarh, India   Rizwan Ahmad Khan
Aligarh, India   Shagufta Wahab

Contents

1 **Introduction and Epidemiology of Abdominal Trauma in Children** 1
Nitin Borkar

2 **Injury and Risk of Abdominal Trauma in Children** 7
Rizwan Ahmad Khan and Shagufta Wahab

3 **Prevention of Paediatric Abdominal Trauma**..................... 11
Neeti Goswami

4 **Post-traumatic Stress Disorder in Children**..................... 19
Deoshree Akhouri

5 **Prehospital and Initial Trauma Care** 31
Nidhi Sugandhi

6 **Assessment of a Child with Abdominal Trauma** 41
Rizwan Ahmad Khan

7 **Imaging in Pediatric Abdominal Trauma**....................... 53
Shagufta Wahab

8 **Interventional Imaging in Pediatric Abdominal Trauma** 67
Shagufta Wahab

9 **Anesthetic and Critical Care Considerations in Children with Abdominal Trauma** 73
Lalit Gupta and Bhavna Gupta

10 **Blunt Solid Organ Injuries in Children** 89
Rizwan Ahmad Khan

11 **Genitourinary Injuries in Pediatric Blunt Trauma** 97
Tanveer Roshan Khan and Rizwan Ahmad Khan

12 Blunt Bowel Injuries in Children 107
Rizwan Ahmad Khan

13 Abdominal Wall Injuries in Blunt Trauma. 113
Manal Mohd Khan

14 Other Blunt Injuries in Children. 121
Rizwan Ahmad Khan and Shagufta Wahab

About the Editors

.

Rizwan Ahmad Khan is an associate professor and head of the Department of Pediatric Surgery, Jawaharlal Nehru Medical College, Aligarh Muslim University, Aligarh. He received his superspecialization in pediatric surgery from the PGI, Chandigarh. His areas of interest are pediatric trauma, pediatric urology including pediatric hernia, hydrocele, undescended testes, ureteropelvic junction obstruction, posterior urethral valves, and congenital hydrocephalus. He has published more than 50 articles in peer-reviewed international and national journals of pediatric surgery and two book chapters. He is a member of various pediatric surgery bodies of India and abroad and serves as a reviewer for many prominent journals of pediatrics.

Shagufta Wahab holds an M.D. in radiodiagnosis and is a consultant radiologist currently working as an associate professor at the Department of Radiodiagnosis, Jawaharlal Nehru Medical College, Aligarh Muslim University, Aligarh. She has published more than 40 papers related to radiodiagnosis in various peer-reviewed national and international journals, as well as a handbook. Her main field of research is pediatric and women's imaging and MRI, with an emphasis on newer techniques like MR spectroscopy, diffusion and perfusion imaging, MR urography, and MR angiography. She is an active member of various international and national radio-logical societies.

Nitin Borkar

1.1 Background and Epidemiology

Epidemiology of paediatric trauma is related to the collection of data in relation to the mechanism of injury, place of injury, demographic details of the victim of the trauma and analysing the data. After analysing the injury epidemiology, it has been identified that trauma is one of the leading causes of morbidity and mortality in the paediatric age group. Children are not just miniature adults. There are anatomical, physiological and emotional variations among children and adults that make the care and management of paediatric population different from that of adult. In 1960 WHO regional office for Europe found that in high- income countries, trauma had become the primary cause of death in children above 1 year of age [1]. The mechanism for paediatric trauma encompasses both intentional and unintentional injuries. Intentional injuries occur because of violence, conflicts, war, suicides and child abuse. Unintentional injuries occur because of the vehicular accident, fall, sport- related injuries, poisoning, burns and drowning. The pattern and cause of paediatric trauma have changed over the period of time with globalisation, urbanisation and motorisation [2]. There is a difference in pattern and cause of injuries in developed and developing country and also between urban and rural area. There are differences in the causes of injuries in the same country with different socioeconomic status and different geographical location. The age group which is kept protected from economical responsibility in one country or one socioeconomic status may be the main contributor for family economy in others that makes them more vulnerable to agent factor of trauma.

The mechanism of injury is also found to be different for different age groups in different socioeconomic status. The agent factors responsible for paediatric trauma have never been studied fully. And at present, there are no injury prevention

N. Borkar
Department of Pediatric Surgery, All India Institute of Medical Sciences, Raipur, India

© Springer Nature Singapore Pte Ltd. 2018   1
R. Ahmad Khan, S. Wahab (eds.), *Blunt Abdominal Trauma in Children*,
https://doi.org/10.1007/978-981-13-0692-1_1

programmes for paediatric population in India and other developing countries as well [3]. One of the major reasons for this lacuna could be the dearth of dedicated trauma centres or dedicated paediatric unit in the existing trauma centres in these countries [4]. Such type of facilities exists in the western world which had contributed to the improved survival of paediatric trauma patients.

1.2   Historical and Social Perspectives

Historically communicable diseases and malnutrition were the leading causes of mortality in the paediatric age group. The advent of immunisation, improvement of social and economic conditions and national programmes targeting infectious diseases and nutritional deficiencies have reduced the incidence of childhood mortality. At the same time, trauma has emerged as the most important causative factor for childhood mortality. Those children who are saved from communicable diseases and malnutrition are becoming victims of trauma. Pizzi [5] in 1968 observed that the margin between survival and death is very narrow in most trauma victims; hence emergency departments must be geared up to widen this margin. For that, he stressed for the care of trauma victims in each phase of emergency from ambulance to operation theatre as well as a team approach in an emergency. The concept of trauma care system and trauma centre was started in reference to the publication of an important US government report in the year 1970 "Accidental Death and Disability: The Neglected Disease of Modern Society", which was prepared by the Committees on Trauma and Shock, Division of Medical Sciences, National Academy of Sciences and National Research Council [6]. The first paediatric trauma centre was established in the United States soon after adult centres in the 1970s and 1980s. Although trauma centres with integrated trauma care are in place in many areas of the United States, only a few dedicated paediatric trauma centres are available to cater all major paediatric trauma cases under one roof [7]. The landmark Convention on the Right of Child was adopted by the United Nations General Assembly on 20 November 1989. One of its article states that "children around the world have a right for the safe environment and to get protection for injury and violence". In 2000 the United Nations resolved to achieve a two-third reduction in the 11 million deaths reported among under-five children by the year 2015. Reduction in deaths due to injury and violence which are the principal cause of death in children over 1 year of age will be an important aspect of achieving this goal [8]. In May 2002, the United Nations General Assembly, in a special session on children and came out with a document: *A World Fit for Children*. One of the specific goals that were adopted in this action plan was to decrease the incidence of child injuries due to accidents or other causes through development and execution of proper preventive measures [9].

Many studies from different countries and also from major cities in India have found that boys are more commonly injured than girls. This may be because boys are given more freedom and opportunities in comparison to girls in our society. Also, they are more exposed to potential risk-taking behaviours like playing on roads and climbing on trees [10].

Nonaccidental trauma is also a major cause morbidity and mortality among children. Though various studies outlined that it accounts for 3–7.3% of all traumatic injuries evaluated at trauma centres, it may still be under-reported [11, 12]. Trauma causes profound unpleasant late effects on the injured children and their families. Even 1 or more years after injury, almost 75% of the children have to contend with disabilities [13]. Effect on family is also striking though sometimes it is difficult to recognise. Relation between the injured child and his siblings and parents becomes more fragile. Changes in psychosocial behaviour of the patient especially after head injury also affect sibling and parents. Family finances also get affected. Sometimes one of the family members has to stop working to take care of the injured child. Sometimes trauma to child can be the cause of marital conflicts between parents. Uninjured siblings also develop some emotional reactions, learning problem and personality changes [13].

It is very difficult to estimate the actual cost to treat paediatric trauma as it not only involves cost of hospitalisation but also involves loss of productivity of families and income. Those patients who underwent major surgical procedure for trauma have more cost of care as compared to those who underwent minor surgical procedure or managed conservatively. There was also a positive correlation between increasing hospital cost and increasing trauma score [14].

1.3   Magnitude of Problem (Morbidity and Mortality)

Paediatric trauma is closely associated with community-based determinants of the society. The saddle of injury in children is unequally distributed in overall world. Children in low-income group of nations and those from poor families in more affluent nations are the most vulnerable lot. More than 95% of deaths due to paediatric trauma are noticed in low-income and middle-income group of nations. Even though the rate of deaths due to paediatric trauma is quite less in developed nations, it accounts for approximately 40% of paediatric mortality in these countries [2].

Paediatric trauma occurs worldwide and is becoming a global health problem. The reasons may be a significant proportion (around half) of worldwide population is now younger than 25 years old and social, economic and technical development has resulted in increased vehicular traffic. Additionally the presence of armed conflicts around the world involves children as innocent victims [15]. Above 1 year of age, trauma is one of the most common causes of mortality. Road traffic accidents are responsible for the loss of around 260,000 children and teenagers each year, i.e. a loss of 718 individuals from the most productive age group per day. Non-fatal trauma events lead to morbidity in further ten million children. The mode of injury and death varies among nations. In developed nations, the most common mechanism of injury and death among children occurs while they are occupants of vehicles. In contrast the children in developing nations suffer injury and deaths usually as pedestrians or while cycling. All over the world, approximately 950,000 deaths occur due to physical violence among children who are in late teens. Ninety percent of these deaths are classified as "unintentional" [2]. Almost half of all the deaths due to unintentional trauma are caused by road traffic accidents and drowning. According to the latest data made available by the Government of India about road accidents, 146,133 deaths and 500,279 injuries occurred due to road accidents in the year 2015. Out of 146,133 persons who died in the accidents, 5937 (4.1%) persons were between the age group of 0–14 years, and 6652 (4.55%) persons were between the age group of 15–17 years. [16]. The National Crime Records Bureau (NCRB) data reveals that out of 413,457 total accidental deaths in the year 2015, 17,861 were between the age group of 0–14 years, and 26,736 were between the age group of 14–18 years. The age group of 0–18 years comprises of 10.7% of total accidental deaths [17]. Accidental fall is also one of the leading causes of presentation of trauma victims to emergency department. Around 47,000 children die due to fall every year. But this is only a tip of iceberg as for each death due to fall, there are another 690 children who either have school time loss or seek treatment and 4 children who suffer from a permanent disability [2].

In 2013 unintentional injuries of all types and penetrating trauma caused 6489 deaths among children in the age group of 1–19 years which represented 34% of all paediatric deaths and a mortality rate of 8.3 per 100,000 per year [18]. According to the data available in CDC for 2015, in the United States, unintentional injuries are the fifth most common cause of death in less than 1-year age group. Between the age group of 1 and 14 years, unintentional injuries are the most common cause of death [19].

Combined result of South and East Asia documented suffocation as the main mode of injury-related death in children less than 1 year of age. Road traffic accident is the most common mode of trauma in boys followed by fall and assault. In contrast to boys, fall is the most common mode of trauma in girls followed by road traffic accident [3]. And the most common area of sustaining fall injuries in girls is at home or at play area. This is followed by fall from roof, stairs, bed or tree [3]. Overall for paediatric injuries, road traffic accident is the commonest cause of death followed by fall-related injuries. Most mortality occurred in polytrauma patients followed by patients with head injuries [20]. The most common category of unintentional injury requiring hospitalisation suffered by children under the age of 15 years is fractured extremities [21].

Each year around ten million children get injured or disabled as a result of road traffic accidents. Data estimate from South-East Asia shows that for every child who dies, there are 254 children who require hospital admission and further management and 4 of these sustain some form of permanent disability. Most common injuries include head injuries and fractured limbs. Around 10–20% of children involved in road traffic crashes sustain multiple injuries [2].

Road traffic injury is a leading cause of permanent disability for children estimating 20 per 100,000 children aged 1–17 years in South-East Asia. Road traffic accident can lead to psychological effect and mental health disorder in children, such as post-traumatic stress disorder. By 2030 it is predicted that road traffic accidents will be the fifth leading cause of death worldwide and the seventh leading cause of Disability-Adjusted Life Years (DALY) lost [2].

1.4   Risk Factors

The increase risk of paediatric injury is associated with single parentage, large family, poorly built houses and parenteral drug abuse. Young maternal age also can increase the risk of paediatric injuries because of her lack of experience and maturity. Stairs, balconies and rooftop without railings and easily accessible, open windows without grills can be the risk factors for fall. Uncovered wells and lack of isolation fencing for kid's swimming pool increase the risk of drowning. Easy accessibility of harmful objects like sharp object and explosives to kids increases the risk of injury due to these objects.

When we consider road traffic injuries, risk factors at host level are male sex and young age. Behavioural issues like substance abuse and high-speed driving also are associated with increased risk of traffic injury. Not wearing safety devices like helmets or seatbelts and the use of devices like mobile phones and headphone while driving also have been linked to higher risk of sustaining road traffic injuries. The lack of driving experience and lack of knowledge about road traffic rules can also lead to higher risks of injury.

At the level of the agent, the lack of safety features such as seatbelts, airbags, child restraint system in car and reverse parking sensor or camera and vehicle size are also related with increased risks of injury. Poorly maintained vehicle with nonfunctional sensors or indicators can be risk to other vehicles leading to injuries. Heavy motor vehicles represent a higher risk for pedestrians and for smaller vehicles. Environmental conditions like traffic congestion, lack of proper signage, mechanised safety barriers and traffic calming devices also contribute to increased risks of trauma.

1.5   Summary

Trauma is emerging as the leading cause of death in paediatric age group. Majority of paediatric injuries are preventable which stress for increased awareness in the society and robust preventive strategies to reduce the incidence of paediatric trauma.

References

1. The prevention of accidents in childhood. Report of a seminar, Spa, Belgium 16–25 July 1958. Copenhagen: World Health Organization Regional Office for Europe; 1960.
2. Peden M, et al., editors. World report on injury prevention. Geneva: World Health Organisation; 2008.
3. Kundal VK, Debnath PR, Sen A. Epidemiology of pediatric trauma and its pattern in urban India: a tertiary care hospital-based experience. JIAPS. 2017;22(1):33–7.
4. WHO/UNICEF. Child and adolescent injury prevention: a global call to action. Geneva: WHO; 2005.
5. Pizzi WF. The management of multiple injury patients. J Trauma. 1968;8(1):91–103.

6. Committee on Trauma and Committee on Shock. Division of Medical Sciences. National Academy of Sciences. National Research Council. Accidental death and disability: the neglected disease of modern society. Public Health Service Publication Number 1071-A-13. Sixth Printing September 1970.

7. Wesson DE. Pediatric trauma centers coming of ages. Tex Heart Inst J. 2012;39:871–3.

8. United Nations Millennium Declaration. New York, NY, United Nations. 2000. (A/RES/55/2). http://www.un.org/millennium/declaration/ares552e.htm.

9. A world fit for children. New York, NY, United Nations General Assembly. 2002. (A/RES/S-27/2). http://www.unicef.org/specialsession/docs_new/documents/A-RES-S27-2E.pdf.

10. Sharma M, Lahoti BK, Khandelwal G, Mathur RK, Sharma SS, Laddha A. Epidemiological trends of pediatric trauma: a single-Centre study of 791patients. JIAPS. 2011;16(3):88–92.

11. Roaten JB, Partrick DA, Nydam TL, Bensard DD, Hendrickson RJ, Sirontak AP, Karrer FM. Nonaccidental trauma is a major cause of morbidity and mortality among patients at a regional level 1 pediatric trauma center. J Pediatr Surg. 2006;41(12):2013–5.

12. Cox CS. Trauma from child abuse. In: Wesson DE, editor. Pediatric trauma. New York: Taylor and Francis; 2006. p. 73.

13. Harris BH, Schwaitzberg SD, Seman TM, Herrmann C. The hidden morbidity of pediatric trauma. J Pediatr Surg. 1989;24(1):103–6.

14. Harris BH, Bass KD, O'Brien MD. Hospital reimbursement for pediatric trauma care. J Pediatric Surg. 1996;31(1):78–80.

15. Sharar SR. The ongoing and worldwide challenge of pediatric trauma. Int J Crit Illn Inj Sci. 2012;2(3):111–3.

16. Road accidents in India. Report by Government of India Ministry of Road Transport and Highways Transport Research Wing; 2015.

17. National Crime Records Bureau Ministry of Home Affairs Government of India. Accidental Deaths and Suicides in India; 2015.

18. Osterman MJK, Kochanek KD, MacDorman MF, Stobino DM, Guyer B. Annual summary of vital statistics: 2012–13. Pediatrics. 2015;135:1115–25.

19. National Centre for Injury prevention and Control (CDC). 10 Leading causes of injury deaths by Age Group Highlighting Violence – Related Injury Deaths, United States. 2015.

20. Simon R, Gilyoma JM, Dass RM, Mchembe MD, Chalya PL. Paediatric injuries at Bugando Medical Centre in Northwestern Tanzania: a prospective review of 150 cases. J Trauma Manag Outcomes. 2013;7:10.

21. The Global Burden of Disease: 2004 Update. World Health Organisation; 2008.

Injury and Risk of Abdominal Trauma in Children

Rizwan Ahmad Khan and Shagufta Wahab

Trauma nowadays accounts for one of the most important causes of childhood mortality. According to a world report by the WHO and UNICEF (United Nations International Children's Emergency Fund) in 2008, every single day, more than 2000 children die because of accidents. Although fractures of limbs and head and neck injuries are most common, around 10% of trauma deaths in childhood are due to abdominal injuries [1–3]. The abdomen can be afflicted in penetrating or blunt manner. There is difference in this data with respect to developed and developing country [3]. Injury pattern in children is governed by age, gender, ethnicity, and socioeconomic status. In children more than 1 year of age, approximately 50% of deaths are due to trauma [1].

In developed countries, road traffic accidents involving children as pedestrians are the most common cause of injury and deaths in children, while in developing countries, falls and road traffic accidents are equally the common cause of pediatric injuries [2].

2.1 Mechanism and Patterns of Pediatric Abdominal Injury

Both intentional and unintentional injuries can afflict the abdomen. Among unintentional injuries, road traffic accidents are the most common form. These include injury due to motor vehicle accidents or those walking along the road [4]. Others include falls and playground injuries. Falls can occur on level ground or from a height as fall from terrace, tree, roofs, or staircase [5]. Farmland injuries can occur

R. A. Khan (✉)
Department of Pediatric Surgery, Jawaharlal Nehru Medical College, AMU, Aligarh, India

S. Wahab
Department of Radiodiagnosis, Jawaharlal Nehru Medical College, AMU, Aligarh, India

© Springer Nature Singapore Pte Ltd. 2018
R. Ahmad Khan, S. Wahab (eds.), *Blunt Abdominal Trauma in Children*,
https://doi.org/10.1007/978-981-13-0692-1_2

as a result of employment of children for sowing and harvesting with agricultural machineries [6].

Road traffic injuries in toddlers result in abdominal injuries more often as they are often restricted by seat belts [7, 8]. Children in motor vehicle accidents appear to suffer more abdominal trauma if using seat belts or other form of restrains. But other injuries become less severe. Abdominal contusion due to seat belt may point toward serious abdominal trauma like small bowel and duodenal injuries, pancreatic injury, or chance fracture of lumbar vertebrae [6]. Airbags which are supposed to prevent from significant injury pose different sort of problems to children. Airbags can set out at speeds of up to 150 mph, causing significant head injury and abrasions to children [6, 7].

Injuries in older children that occur while they are running across the road cause multiple injuries, usually head and extremities, while abdominal injuries account for only 10% injuries. Abdominal injuries due to bicycle ride in children are difficult to diagnose as the handlebar injury appears insignificant initially [1, 2]. Traumatic pancreatitis is the most common injury followed by renal and splenic trauma and duodenal injuries. It may also be associated with extremity and neck fractures.

Waddell's triad refers to the pattern of injury seen in pedestrian children with a lower limb injury and abdominal or chest injury on the same side as a result of first collision and after the child is thrown over the car, wherein the head strikes the road, causing a contralateral head injury [8, 9].

2.1.1 Age

Children under 4 years old are most commonly afflicted with abdominal injuries which are unintentional, by the mistake of caregiver and natural disasters. The other mechanisms can be child abuse and child restraint in vehicle. The injuries mostly affect the head, cervical spine, and face. Abdominal injury can occur in falls and vehicular accidents.

The children between 5 and 9 years of age suffer significant injuries whatever may be the mechanism of injury. In this age group, also the most common form of injury is head injury. But this is the age group where the abdominal injury is seen most commonly [5, 7]. The children in 10–15-year age group mostly suffer from vehicular accidents, and head and extremity injury are most common.

2.1.2 Gender

The available data on child injuries indicates that beyond 2 years of age, boys experience more injuries than girls. This gender difference is due to higher impulsivity, activity, and socialization levels in boys as compared to girls of the same age [8, 10]. This is compounded by the fact that the risk-taking behavior of boys is not discouraged by the parents as well. The data indicate that the injuries are about two times more common in boys as compared to girls.

2.1.3   Socioeconomic Status

The lower socioeconomic status is associated with risks of falls, road traffic accidents, abuse, and assaults. There is higher incidence of injuries in lower socioeconomic status due to higher traffic volumes; faster vehicle speeds; less use of head gear; poor parental supervision; poor educational status; unfavorable housing designs; low parental health education and adoptive measures; higher, multifactorial exposure to risks in poor areas; poor medical facilities; alcohol and drug abuse; and agricultural setup (associated with three to four times more likelihood of risk of injury) [5, 6, 8]. There is growing evidence that better educational profile and socioeconomic status of parents are associated with better health and growth of their children.

2.1.4   Other Risk Factors

Lack of awareness and education of traffic rules, widespread use of mobiles, and texting while driving also are associated with increased risk of road traffic injuries. Lack of experience, drugs, and alcohol in younger population also contribute to increased risks of injury [6].

The increase risk of pediatric injury is associated with single parentage, large family, poorly built houses, and parenteral drug abuse [7]. Young maternal age also can increase the risk of pediatric injuries because of her lack of experience and maturity. Stairs, balconies, and rooftop without railings and easily accessible, open windows without grills can be the risk factors for fall.

Poor infrastructure and roads, old poor condition vehicles, and non-compliance of traffic norms also contribute to increased road traffic accidents in developing countries.

References

1. Rowe MI, O'Neill JA, Grosfeld JL, Fonkalsrud EW, Coran AG. The injured child. In: Rowe MI, O'Neill JA, Grosfeld JR, Fonkalsrud EW, Coran AG, editors. Essentials of pediatric surgery. St Louis: Mosby; 1996. p. 183–9.
2. Molcho M, Walsh S, Donnelly P, Matos MG, Pickett W. Trend in injury related mortality and morbidity among adolescents across 30 countries from 2002 to 2010. Eur J Pub Health. 2015;25(Suppl 2):33–6.
3. Karbakhsh M, Zargar M, Zarei MR, Khaji A. Childhood injuries in Tehran: a review of 1281 cases. Turk J Pediatr. 2008;50:317–25.
4. Ameh EA, Mshelbwala PM. Challenges of managing paediatric abdominal trauma in a Nigerian setting. Eur J Pediatr Surg. 2007;2:90–5.
5. Simon R, Gilyoma JM, Dass RM, Mchembe MD, Chalya PL. Paediatric injuries at Bugando Medical Centre in Northwestern Tanzania: a prospective review of 150 cases. J Trauma Manag Outcomes. 2013;7:10.
6. Dischinger PC, Cushing BM, et al. Injury patterns associated with direction of impact: drivers admitted to trauma centers. J Trauma. 1993;35:454–9.

7. Adesunkanmi ARK, Oginni LM, Oyelami AO, Badru OS. Epidemiology of childhood injury. J Trauma. 1998;44(3):506–11.
8. Hyder AA, Labinjo M, Muzaffer SSF. A new challenge to child and adolescent survival in urban Africa: an increasing burden of road traffic injuries. Traffic Inj Prev. 2006;7(4):381–8.
9. Solagberu BA. Trauma deaths in children: a preliminary report. Nig J Surg Res. 2002;4(3):98–102.
10. Bahebeck J, Atangana R, Mboudou E, Nonga BN, Sosso M, Malonga E. Incidence, case fatality rate and clinical pattern of firearm injuries in two cities where arm owning is forbidden. Injury. 2005;36:714–7.

Prevention of Paediatric Abdominal Trauma

Neeti Goswami

Injuries have been long perceived as unavoidable happening or accidents which are thus unpredictable and unpreventable. A scientific and logically based approach to prevention has evolved only on later part of the nineteenth century which signifies that injury events can be studied, understood and prevented and therefore are not inevitable as commonly suggested.

Definitions advocated by WHO in field of injury prevention are [1]:
(a) Injury prevention refers to the actions or interventions that prevent an injury event or violent act from happening by rendering it impossible or less likely to occur.
(b) Injury control refers to actions aimed at reducing injuries or the consequences of injuries once they have occurred.

WHO report [2] on child injury reported higher burden of injuries in children of third world countries and those from poorer background in developed countries. Lack of adequate attention to child injuries results in low- and middle-income countries contributing to 95% of all child injury deaths and about 40% child deaths in high-income countries.

Paediatric blunt abdominal trauma resulting in intra-abdominal injury (IAI) may occur due to various causes such as isolated, high-energy blows to the abdomen in case of fall from a bicycle or high-risk trauma mechanisms such as road traffic accidents or falls from height. Table 3.1 describes various blunt trauma mechanisms associated with a high risk of injury in children.

N. Goswami
Community Medicine, All India Institute of Medical Sciences, Jodhpur, India

© Springer Nature Singapore Pte Ltd. 2018
R. Ahmad Khan, S. Wahab (eds.), *Blunt Abdominal Trauma in Children*,
https://doi.org/10.1007/978-981-13-0692-1_3

Table 3.1 Blunt trauma mechanisms associated with a high risk of injury in children

A. Motor vehicle collision
– Throwing out from the vehicle
– Mortality of a co-passenger in the vehicle
– Vehicle roll over
– High-speed automobile crash
(a) Travelling speed >40 mph (64 kph)
(b) Vehicular distortion >20 in. (50 cm)
(c) Incursion of vehicle body into passenger area >12 in. (30 cm)
– Extrication time >20 min
– Motorbike crash at >20 mph (32 kph) or associated with throwing of the rider
B. Motor vehicle-pedestrian injury
– Pedestrian thrown or run over
– Automobile-pedestrian injury at >5 mph (8 kph) collision
C. Falls
– Child: >10 ft. (3 m) or more than 2–3 times patient height

3.1   Basics of Injury Prevention

As illustrated by Heinrich's "injury pyramid" [3], the burden of paediatric deaths due to blunt abdominal trauma represents only a small fraction of those injured. A large proportion of affected paediatric population is reflected in form of emergency department visits, hospitalization records, consultations to general physicians or informal or alternative medical care providers. The severity of injury cases assessed through conventional injury pyramid is further influenced by quality of healthcare services available and the level of injury surveillance system in place.

3.2   Injury Pyramid (Diagram): Burden of Paediatric Injuries on the Healthcare System

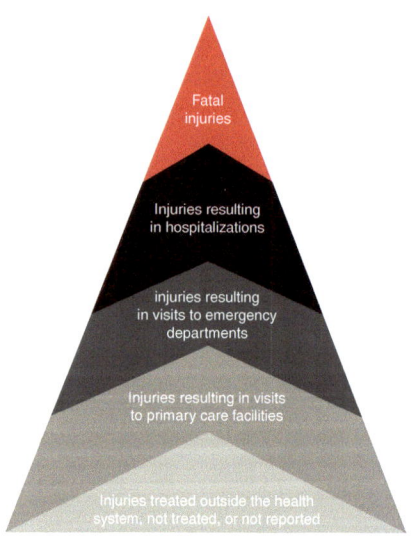

3.3   Public Health Model of Injury Prevention

The public health approach advocates multidisciplinary approach engaging all relevant sectors, disciplines and actors through logical mechanism. Traditionally, all prevention efforts are characterized at three levels and integrate temporal aspect to epidemiological model of diseases. Haddon illustrated this approach in the form of Haddon matrix where vector, host and environment risk factors are identified for an injury contributing towards before, during and after phase of an injury event. Prevention strategies to be operationalized at each of these three stages are described in the form of primary, secondary and tertiary prevention.

Types of Injury Prevention
(a) Primary prevention (pre-event): The steps of prevention are designed at preventing occurrence of injury incidents, e.g. speed limit in residential areas.
(b) Secondary prevention (event): The steps are aimed at minimizing the damage resulting from an injury, e.g. protection of motor cycle rider by using helmet.
(c) Tertiary prevention (post-event): The steps are aimed at treatment and rehabilitation of the injured children, e.g. paediatric trauma specialized units and specialists.

3.3.1   Haddon Illustration of an Injury Event

As per Haddon's definition, injury takes place when energy is transmitted in such amounts and at such quick rates that host/child gets injured. The pre-existing conditions and set of circumstances which can prevent, aggravate or reduce the impact of injury are explained in the form of chain of events occurring at different phases and due to different contributors in the form of Haddon matrix. Such temporal delineation enables better understanding of the impact caused due to causal factor in context of other contributing factors.

The temporal relations of primary, secondary and tertiary phases are graphed alongside the host/person and environmental factors. In this plotted graph, a 12-cell matrix is created by combination of these two axes. This 12-cell matrix is popularly known as Haddon matrix. This model helps in understanding different points of intervention that can be planned to avert or decrease the severity and effect of injuries.

Table 3.2 illustrates the communication of three factors—human being, vector and surroundings—during three phases of a fall event: pre-event, the event and post-event. Based on emergency department and hospital reports all over the world, falls are commonly reported injuries in children requiring hospital care [4, 5]. Reported evidence states that children less than 5 years of age constitute the majority of these patients and home represents one of the major site of incident probably reflecting

Table 3.2 Haddon matrix evaluation for understanding epidemiology of paediatric abdominal injuries due to falls

	Host	Vector	Physical environment	Social environment
Pre-event	– Parent characteristics	– Lack of stair gates, window guards	– Multilevel, low-income, poorly maintained housing – Free and open access to balconies, terraces – Absence of protective parapet on staircase, flyovers	– Lack of building code regulations for windows or window guards [8] and stair gates – Provision of safe ground-level playing areas – Regular playground inspections
Event	– Unsupervised at the time of the fall [9]	– Height of fall/ height of playground equipment – Unsafe playground surfaces (lack of loose fill materials and synthetic rubber mats)	– Easily accessible opening more than 4 in. [10] – Fall on asphalt, concrete, grass and soil surfaces (hard/unforgiving surfaces)	– Inaccessible or poor awareness about accessible and available paediatric emergency care services
Post-event	– Parent's or caretaker ability to communicate with paediatric emergency services	– Presence of hazards (e.g. exposed concrete footings, tree stumps and rocks) around place of fall	– Lack of accessibility for emergency vehicles	– Lack of paediatric emergency health facilities or concerned specialists
Prevention strategies	Active intervention: those where an individual's behaviour is involved (e.g. supervision of children while playing). Such interventions require human involvement for their implementation and results		Passive intervention: aimed at preventing injuries where the individual action is not required (e.g. building code regulations mandating stair gates and window guards)	

the length of time a child spends there [6]. Abdominal injury is likely to occur due to low-level falls in children, while high-level falls are observed to frequently cause head, orthopaedic and thoracic injuries [7].

The public health model advocates informed approach towards injuries aiming to reduce the collective costs and impacts of health problem. Four essential components involved are:

1. Surveillance—to detect the magnitude and proportion of the problem
2. Research—an examination of the risk factors and the causes of the problem
3. Evaluation—finding out ways and strategies for prevention
4. Implementation—introducing prevention programmes on a large scale

3.3.1.1 Injury Surveillance

The cornerstone in formulating effective prevention strategies is robust information system at global, national and local level to know about the nature of injuries that occur, the population subgroup most vulnerable and about the circumstances in which those injuries occur. The public health surveillance is aimed at continuous and organized compilation as well as examination, elucidation and propagation of the findings on health-related issues for utilization in drafting of community action plans so as to decrease the morbidity and mortality thereby leading to overall advancement of community health parameters [11]. Thus, injury surveillance is instrumental in defining the burden at hand and monitoring all facets of the problem. This enables understanding about multiple aspects of paediatric blunt abdominal trauma such as who is at risk, what are the risks, when the problem is likely to occur and where.

Sources of injury surveillance [12]	Records	Indicators
1. Individuals	1. Death certificates	1. Premature mortality
2. Health system	2. Medical examiner or coroner records	2. Preventable morbidity
3. Police records	3. Hospital inpatient and discharge records	3. Description of injuries
4. Fire department	4. Emergency medical records	4. Circumstances and place of incident
5. Insurance agencies	5. Trauma registries	5. Intent of injury
	6. Outpatient care records	6. Pre-injury risk or protective factors

1. Research: Research studies and surveys enable capturing of complete and overall scenario of the occurrence of injuries, the risk factors and the longer-term health consequences of identified health problem. Experimental scientific studies can generate evidence and enable stakeholders to identify cost-effective strategies in tackling the problem. This contributes by identifying the specific risk and protective factors at the individual, community and broad societal levels and explains higher susceptibility of certain communities and age groups as compared to others. As illustrated in Haddon matrix, intervention strategies can be categorized as active and passive intervention. These interventions are further classified as primordial, primary, secondary and tertiary prevention according to the temporal context.

2. Evaluation: The process of evaluation tests multiple aspects of planned intervention. Resources in terms of time, money, human resources and politics determine the level of effectiveness of strategies planned for the target group. Programme evaluation is defined as the "systematic assessment of the processes and/or outcomes of a program with the intent of furthering its development and improvement" [13]. This is essential to understand the facilitating factors and barriers that may likely influence the programme when implemented at larger scale and the expected outcomes that can be intended.

3. Implementation: Strategies at mass level with proven benefits in controlled or clinical settings may prove to be unsuitable, difficult or get plagued by multiple operational factors at field level. Thus, understanding the science behind implementation of cost-effective programme strategies across multiple settings and creating generalizable knowledge is essential. This requires analysis of biological, social and environmental factors which are likely to affect and impact community-wide implementation.

3.3.2   Childhood Injuries: Global Initiatives

Globally, the World Health Organization and United Nations General Assembly have prioritized injury prevention in children in multiple ways. These schemes have emphasized injuries as a community health problem of priority and offer a strategic proposal for enabling an organized and synchronized approach to preventing accidents and injuries in children. Box 3.1 outlines the resolutions adopted by international agencies to prevent childhood injuries.

Box 3.1 Outlining the Resolutions Adopted by Different International Agencies to Prevent Childhood Injuries

Sustainable development goals: goal on prevention of injuries [14]

Goal 3.2—To bring down the neonatal mortality to <12 per 1000 live births and under-5 mortality to <25 per 1000 live births by eliminating the preventable deaths in these age groups till the year 2030

Goal 3.6—To reduce the mortality from injuries from road traffic accidents by 50% till the year 2020

Goal 11.2—To provide access to secure, inexpensive, sustainable conveyance systems and improved road safety for all with particular consideration to the requirements of vulnerable like children, females, elderly and differently abled people

WHO and UN resolution

1. WHA49.25: prevention of violence—a public health priority
2. WHA56.24: implementing the recommendations of the world report on violence and health
3. WHA57.10: road safety and health
4. United Nations General Assembly resolution 58/289: improving global road safety
5. *World report on road traffic injury prevention*, including a manual seat belts and child restraints (2009)

6. WHA58.23: reduction of risk factors contributing to disabilities in childhood
7. *Convention on the Rights of the Child (1989)*: ensure safety in the care and protection of children

Special initiatives by countries

1. CEHAPE (Children's Environment and Health Action Plan for Europe): It is an action plan launched by regional committee resolution (EUR/RC54/R3) (CEHAPE) with a goal of preventing injuries in children but with regional priority [15].
2. Another resolution by the regional committee (EUR/ RC55/R9) aims at prevention of injuries in the European region.
3. *Safe Kids Worldwide "Walk This Way" programme* is a child safety programme backed by FedEx Express. This programme has been extended to nine more countries, including India (2009). It aims to keep child pedestrians safe from injuries through multi-pronged approach like raising awareness, creating safer environments through infrastructure improvements, influencing community-based guidelines and providing road safety education to children beginning from early stage.

References

1. World Health Organization. TEACH-VIP 2 users' manual – training, educating and advancing collaboration in health on violence, and injury prevention – user's manual. Geneva. 2012. Retrieved from www.who.int/violence_injury_prevention/capacitybuilding/teach_vip/en/index.html.
2. WHO. World report on child injury prevention. Geneva: WHO; 2008.
3. Heinrich HW, Petersen D, Roos N. Industrial accident prevention. New York: McGraw-Hill; 1980.
4. Zuckerbraun NS, Powell EC, Sheehan KM, et al. Community childhood injury surveillance: an emergency department-based model. Pediatr Emerg Care. 2004;20:361.
5. Agran PF, Anderson C, Winn D, et al. Rates of pediatric injuries by 3-month intervals for children 0 to 3 years of age. Pediatrics. 2003;111:e683.
6. Mathers LJ, Weiss HB. Incidence and characteristics of fall-related emergency department visits. Acad Emerg Med. 1998;5:1064.
7. Wang MY, Kim KA, Griffith PM, et al. Injuries from falls in the pediatric population: an analysis of 729 cases. J Pediatr Surg. 2001;36:1528.
8. Lehman D, Schonfeld N. Falls from heights: a problem not just in the northeast. Pediatrics. 1993;92:121.
9. Harris VA, Rochette LM, Smith GA. Pediatric injuries attributable to falls from windows in the United States in 1990–2008. Pediatrics. 2011;128:455.
10. Committee on Injury and Poison Prevention. American Academy of Pediatrics. Falls from heights: windows, roofs, and balconies. Pediatrics. 2001;107:1188.

11. German RR, Lee LM, Horan JM, Milstein RL, Pertowski CA, Waller MN, Guidelines Working Group Centers for Disease Control and Prevention (CDC). Updated guidelines for evaluating public health surveillance systems: recommendations from the guidelines working group. MMWR Recomm Rep. 2001;50(RR–13):1–51. http://www.cdc.gov/mmwr/PDF/RR/RR5013.pdf

12. Horan JM, Mallonee S. Injury surveillance. Epidemiol Rev. 2003;25(1):24–42. https://doi.org/10.1093/epirev/mxg010

13. Rossi PH, Freeman HE. Evaluation: a systematic approach. 5th ed. Newbury Park: Sage Publications, Inc.; 1993.

14. United Nations. Transforming our world: the 2030 Agenda for Sustainable Development. 2015. http://www.un.org/ga/search/view_doc.asp?symbol=A/RES/70/1&Lang=E.

15. WHO Europe. Regional Committee for Europe Fifty-fourth session. 2004. Accessed from http://www.euro.who.int/__data/assets/pdf_file/0003/88275/RC54_eres03.pdf.

Post-traumatic Stress Disorder in Children

4

Deoshree Akhouri

The purpose of this chapter is to emphasize the effect of trauma on children and its psychological treatment and rehabilitation. Traumatic accidents suffered by children of 0–6 years of age are referred to as early childhood trauma. About one million children are exposed to psychological stress due to trauma every year, e.g., disasters, life-threatening accidents, amputation, etc. Psychological squeal is caused by permanent physical damage or disability due to serious injuries known as traumatic amputations [1]. Trauma directly affects the child's as well as family member's emotional and behavioral well-being. Post-traumatic stress disorder (PTSD) is caused by different types of transient or chronic physical, behavioral, or emotional problem which takes place due to psychological trauma in children. Children susceptible to trauma develop psychiatric disorders particularly anxiety and depression.

According to the American Psychiatric Association's current definition, which was introduced in 1994, post-traumatic stress disorder is a state where an individual should have undergone or observed an incident or collection of incidents which implicated factual or impended fatality or solemn damage or forebode physical probity of oneself or someone else, involving fright, powerlessness, and consternation [2]. Trauma is a state when someone has come across an uncontrollable, terrifying occurrence that has detached oneself from all sense of handling resourcefulness, security, or love [3].

Sufferings in the form of lancinations, lesion and severe sickness, and encroaching medical subroutine such as operations or medicamentations (like burn care) which could be alarming tend to have reaction from ward and their guardians, hence being referred to as pediatric medical traumatic stress [4]. The reaction tends to afflict the body along with the mind. For instance, wards and their guardians might portray apprehensiveness or cranky behavior. They,

D. Akhouri
Department of Psychiatry, AMU, Aligarh, India

© Springer Nature Singapore Pte Ltd. 2018
R. Ahmad Khan, S. Wahab (eds.), *Blunt Abdominal Trauma in Children*,
https://doi.org/10.1007/978-981-13-0692-1_4

children and their families alike, might experience cognitive distortion (irrational speculations) or ordeal about sickness, lesion, or infirmary stay. They might show low interest in social contact with friends and family and may even lose interest in pleasurable activities. Such behaviors may also affect their school performance and personal life. Reactions or improvement can vary from person to person because of their personal opinions or intuitions about sickness, lesion, or infirmary. Memories connected with shock/trauma are tacit and neutralize recollection which still can be initiated by precipitant from the in vivo surroundings. An individual's responses to unenclosed specifications of shocking incident include fright and powerlessness, which are apparent as confused or tremulous behavior in children [5, 6].

The chief reason of fatal death and disablement in children are pediatric injuries. Nearly five million children pass away from trauma each year according to Holder et al. [7]. The National Crime Records Bureau (NCRB) statistics showed that nearly 15–20% of trauma deaths happen among children. In 2006, NCRB reported that there were approximately 22,000 deaths in the age group of less than 14 years because of injuries. The developing countries happen to have few such cases showing the prevalence and potential risk factors of pediatric trauma. It has been evaluated that one in four children undergoes accidental injuries which need medical care yearly. Millions of children are in need of infirmary care each year for nonfatal injury. Injuries related to child disabilities are mostly caused by road traffic accidents and fall. The significant burden of psychological stress disorders, of 95% of child's injuries, happens in low- and middle-income countries of pediatric age group following trauma.

After head injury, many victims developed psychological problems. Due to severe head injury, sufferers' personality changed dramatically. In this condition family members are not able to cope with this situation. They themselves develop psychological problem and need psychological help. First public outing is very scary for victims (e.g., acid attacks, amputation, burns, and physical injuries). Victims need to focus on the possibilities of the moment, present and future, and should let go of the past for the change. Living the life in the moment and present will help the victim in accepting the change and making their life beautiful [8].

Up to now, there is no community-centered epidemiological study which has analyzed extensive presence of PTSD among children. Nevertheless, studies have shown that children who have had experiences of traumatic incidents precisely such as accidents, abuse, or natural disasters are under high risk of prevalence of PTSD. The data of the National Survey of Adolescents was done by Kilpatrick and colleagues (2003) involving data of 4023 patients (between 12 and 17 years of age) for assessing the prevalence of PTSD among adolescents [9]. The 6-month prevalence of PTSD was seen to be 3.7% for boys and 6.3% for girls under the method of DSM-IV criteria. PTSD is more likely to be developed in people who have experienced interpersonal trauma (for instance, assault or child abuse) rather than those who witnessed other forms of trauma like accidents [10]. It has been noted by multiple researchers that when symptoms of post-traumatic stress occur once, it leads to neurophysiologic development in children and adolescents [10].

Child sexual abuse is a universal problem, and it is a fact that millions of girls and boys worldwide are being sexually assaulted within family and outside. Childhood sexual abuse often causes adult PTSD. Molestation can damage the child's growth, boundaries, and self-esteem. Wyatt et al. [11] found that lifetime rates of PTSD in women were significantly higher for those who had histories of childhood sexual abuse [11].

The sexual abuse in a child is defined as any act of abnormal contact between an adult and a child. This includes consensual sexual intercourse, nonconsensual sex (rape), incest, oral sex, etc. Any person can be sexual child abusers whether it is father, mother, relatives, siblings, babysitters, teachers, or strangers. Sexually abused children's behavior and emotion get considerable change. The changes noticed are mainly seductive behavior, averting talks related to sexuality or denunciation of own genitalia, unwarranted violent behavior, and apprehension of a particular individual or member of the family. They often experience uncontrolled emotion, and sometimes they become angry and attacking. Studies have found that fear is a common emotion among both women and men who have histories of sexual abuse. Lobel [12] established that 63% of females who had a history of sexual abuse during childhood testified guilt, worthlessness, and self-hatred [12].

The parliament of India approved the "Protection of Children from Sexual Offences Act, 2012" (POCSO [13]). This act has been implemented with effect from 14 November 2012 in all Indian states except Jammu and Kashmir. This act has toughened the legal stand against the perpetrators of sexual abuse and exploitation in children [13, 14].

4.1 Diagnosis

The official introduction of the new diagnosis of PTSD was in 1980 in the revised version of DSM-III. Later on, features specific to PTSD in children were added in DSM-111-R. The trauma and stress or related disorders include PTSD in DSM-V (2013). PTSD diagnostic criteria has been discussed in 309.81 (F43.10) in DSM-V [15–19].

There are seven precise diagnostic criteria in children aged 6 years or younger of PTSD which have been listed in DSM-V.

The exposure to factual or impended death, severe lesion, or sexual violation in one or in excess of the following manners fall under the first criteria:

- Traumatic event(s) being witnessed directly
- Witnessing of event(s) in-person as it occurred to someone else, especially primary caretakers

The second criterion adheres to the presence of one or more of the following interference symptoms in connection with the traumatic event, which begins after the event occurred:

- The upsetting recollections of the traumatic event(s) are involuntary, recurrent, and disturbing: these recollections may be expressed as play reenactment rather than appearing as necessarily distressing.
- Recurrence of distressing dreams whose content or affect of the content is related to traumatic event(s): to establish the idea that the fear-provoking content is related to traumatic event(s) might not be possible.
- If the child behaves or acts as if the traumatic event(s) were recurring, it might be in the condition of dissociative reactions (e.g., flashbacks or hallucinations): trauma-specific reenactment during play might be carried out by children.
- The exposures of internal or external happening that symbolizes or looks alike to any aspect of traumatic event(s) have intense or prolonged psychological distress.
- The traumatic event(s) are marked by psychological reactions as reminders.

The presence of one or more of the following symptoms represents either pessimistic change in cognition and frame of mind or constant evasion of stimuli linked with traumatic event(s) under third criteria which begins after the event(s) or after worsening of it:

Continuous evasion of stimuli
- Efforts to evade actions, places, or objective reminder that enhance recollection of the distressing event(s)
- Efforts to evade people, discussions, or interpersonal circumstances which may enhance memories of traumatic event(s)

Negative changes in cognition
- Augmented frequencies of pessimistic emotional conditions, e.g., fright, guiltiness, depression, humiliation, and confusion
- Prominent loss of interest in important activities, e.g., decreased interest in play
- Antisocial activities
- Continuous decrease in expressing optimistic sentiments

The change in stimulation and response connected with the traumatic event(s) from the start or deterioration after traumatic event(s) falls in the fourth criterion. It is evidenced by two or more of the following:

- Verbal or physical aggression toward people with extreme temper tantrums shown by imitable behavior and angry outburst
- Hypervigilance
- Exaggerated response of being surprised

- Concentration problems
- Sleep disturbance (e.g., insomnia or sleepiness or restlessness during sleep)

The fifth criterion runs on the condition that the period of the disorder must extend 1 month.

The clinically important distress or changes in relationships with siblings, parents, contemporaries, or other caretakers or in school behavior caused by the disturbance fall under the category of sixth criteria.

The seventh and final criteria states that the impairment cannot be assigned to the pathophysiological effects of a substance, e.g., drugs, alcohol, or other infirmary conditions.

The following are the additional specifiers:

- Depersonalization: recurrence of experiences of feeling disconnected and as an external spectator of one's psychological practices or body, such as feeling of dreamfulness, a sense of nonexistence of the self, or the slow moving time
- Derealization: recurrence of experiences of unreal surroundings (e.g., the individual witnesses the world as unreal, dreamlike, or far away)

In nutshell, symptoms of shock can be said to be of physical, cognitive, behavioral, and emotional in nature. In physical/environmental symptoms, excessive alertness, fatigue/exhaustion, disturbed sleep, etc. are involved, whereas cognitive symptoms include intrusive thought and memory of the incident, nightmares, lack of concentration, and confusion. In behavioral symptoms, there is distance from places or activities that act as reminders of the incident, isolation or anti-social behavior, and lack of interest in any activity. Emotional symptoms involve fright, anger, irritability, guilt, numbness, isolation, anxiety, and horror.

4.2 Assessment

Long-term skilled care is needed for people who survived childhood trauma and might suffer lifelong disability. Chronic physical problems in a child may transform into a chronically ill adult. Unique challenges are presented in the evaluation and management of traumatized children and adolescents for PTSD. Since chronic course of PTSD can disrupt emotional development, it becomes difficult to evaluate a child or an adolescent. The healing process is never simple for a survivor [17]. The American Academy of Child and Adolescent Psychiatry (AACAP) made three major recommendations for the assessment of PTSD in children and adolescents which were published in "Practice Parameters for the Assessment and Treatment of Children and Adolescents with Post Traumatic Stress Disorder":

1. Usage of clinical interview with special focus on PTSD symptoms
2. Developmental influences recognition
3. Implementing trauma-focused treatment interventions

The clinical psychologists play significant role in the smooth recovery of children, adolescents, and families after distressing incidents. Mental health professionals may help in reducing stress and support the patient, family, and public by clarification on their existing strengths and assets. In order to reduce stress of children and their families, specific problem-solving support is much needed equipment, because due to excessive stress individuals fail to use their original methods of survival. For different times and different levels of severity of symptoms, different strategies are opted, such as supportive and problem-focused approach in acute phase of recovery in case of children who suffer distress immediately after the accident. However, if the same level of distress is shown by child later on, more intensive, problem-focused approach is needed. In short-term trauma therapy, a patient may experience it as an immediate result of a traumatic event. Victims need emergency trauma counseling in an accident, natural catastrophe, or sudden loss. Trauma therapy is planned to help a patient to cope with the first shock and pain of an event or experience. It is not planned as a long term, but it is an effective emergency treatment for patient to give the best chance for their later healing. Long-term trauma therapy can help in severe reaction that can have a major effect on the life of a victim. Depending on severity of the trauma, PTS can trigger panic attack, anger, depression, social withdrawal, sexual dysfunction, etc. Asking directly and obtaining assessment of their own symptoms are supposed to be good practice to evaluate anxiety and depression among children.

Before planning therapy it is necessary to know the level of severity of the client. It is helpful for the therapist to plan which therapy is necessary for the victim. It is also helpful to know the improvement after therapy. There are different kinds of assessment tools for PTSD in children and adolescent. These are:

1. Clinician-Administered PTSD Scale for Children and Adolescents for DSM-IV (CAPS—CA [17]) is a detailed, structured clinical interview which was developed by the National Center for PTSD and the University of California, Los Angeles Trauma Psychiatry Program. In October 1998 for DSM-IV criteria, CAPS-CA was revised [18].

2. Children's PTSD Inventory (CPTSDI [20]) is a rapidly administered interview developed to assess for PTSD for individuals between 7 and 18 of age. The CPTSDI includes five possible diagnoses: no PTSD, acute PTSD, chronic PTSD, delayed-onset PTSD, and no diagnosis. Inventory administration requires between 5 and 20 min depending on the trauma history of the child [20].

3. To assess trauma severity, the Injury Severity Score (ISS) which is associated with mortality, morbidity, and length of hospital stay after trauma is used to describe the grades of trauma. If ISS is >15, it is defined as major trauma or polytrauma. The range of ISS is from 1 to 75, i.e., score of 5 for each category [21].

4. The Pediatric Glasgow Coma Scale (ORG [22]) is used to assess the mental state of child patients which is equivalent of Glasgow Coma Scale (GCS). GCS was modified to form the PGCS as many of the assessments for adults would not be

applicable to children. The PGCS comprises three variables: eye, verbal, and motor responses. The lowest possible PGCS is 3 (deep coma or death), and the highest is 15 (fully awake and aware person) [22].

5. Child Post-traumatic Stress Reaction Index (CPTS-RI) is the most widely used tool for assessing PTSD in children. It consists of 20 items, and measure can be used as a self-report instrument for both older children and adolescents. Semi-structured interview is applied on younger children. Administration of the CPTS-RI takes 20–45 min.

    The self-report format is suitable for children at least 8 years of age, and no minimum age is given for the semi-structured format. The possible score range is 0–80 in which scores less than 7 are no PTSD, scores 7–9 are mild PTSD, scores 10–12 are moderate PTSD, and scores greater than 12 are classified as severe PTSD.

6. Trauma Symptom Checklist for Children (TSCC [5]) is a homogeneous test of children aged 7–17 from diverse racial, economic, and regional backgrounds. The TSCC is appropriate for children ages from 8 to 16. This test has two forms. This checklist consists 54 items. Each variable of the TSCC is measured or recorded on a four-point scale, ranging from 0 to 3.

7. Center for Epidemiological Studies Depression Scale has been modified to Center for Epidemiological Studies Depression Scale for Children which measures and assesses both negative symptoms and improvement in symptoms in children of age 6–17 years. It is a 20-point self-recording depression list with scores ranging from 0 to 60. CES-DC was originally designed to gauge the prevalence depression among children and adolescents in extensive epidemiological studies. The score of 15 is indicative of depression in children and adolescents. CES-DC is a consistent and applicable measure of symptoms of depression in children.

4.3 Management

Today mental health professionals play significant role in treating real and painful effects of PTSD. It is treated by a variety of forms of psychotherapy and pharmacotherapy. There are number of therapies for PTSD.

There are some processes involved in trauma therapy.

1. Psychoeducation: information regarding trauma and developmentally appropriate expectations for children and adolescents, course, prognosis, prevalence of illness, and education of vulnerabilities and various adaptable coping mechanisms.

2. ER (emotional regulation) means proper regulation of one's emotions, and it is a process involving the initiating, inhibiting, and grounding of feelings and sentiments from inner creation to an outer depiction and modulating certain aspects of functioning: (a) subjective experience of emotion (internal feeling states), (b) emotions related to cognition (reactions to situations), (c) emotional physiological

processes (hormonal changes), and (d) emotions related to behavior (facial expression).

3. Cognitive processing: depressing insight and thoughts are transformed to optimistic ones about self, others, and surroundings.
4. Trauma processing: includes response activation, counter-conditioning and systematic desensitization, and resolution from traumatic event (state where relief is expressed and stress is not triggered).
5. Emotional processing: involves reconstruction of beliefs, perceptions, and invalid prospects when trauma-related uncertainties are self-activated and familiarized in new life contexts causing predicament of feelings.
6. Experiential processing: involves relief state and methods of relaxation.

Some important therapies which are widely used for PTSD are:

4.3.1 Psychological First Aid/Crisis Intervention

The National Child Traumatic Stress Network and National Center for PTSD [16] developed Psychological First Aid in America. Crisis intervention is an urgent and acute psychological intervention after trauma. It mainly works to alleviate minor distress, stabilize emotion, and regain adaptation of victims and family members. The onset of stress and trauma-related disorders is prevented and reduced in the initial distress caused by traumatic events.

The Red Cross and WHO and Red Crescent Society recommended PFA strongly on humanitarian grounds [23].

4.3.2 Trauma-Focused Cognitive Behavior Therapy

It has its focus on painful and intrusive patterns of behavior by teaching survivors of PTSD. In preventing PTSD and reducing depressive symptoms, CBT is more effective. Brief TF-CBT uses psychoeducation as a method for traumatic reactions (e.g., sadness, anger, guilt); relaxation training, imagery exposure, and in vivo exposure techniques decrease evasion manners and increase feeling of control of personal experiences [24].

4.3.3 Eye Movement Desensitization and Reprocessing (EMDR)

EMD technique was first proposed by Shapiro in 1989 for victims to desensitize the memory from trauma and improve their cognitive function. EMDR aims to lessen the long-term effects of recollections related to distressing events by involving the brain's normal adaptive information processing mechanisms. The use of EMDR in the management of children who have undergone a traumatic event has been found to be quite beneficial. Eye movements or other types of left-right stimulus can "unfreeze" traumatic memories. The precedent, current, and prospective aspects of a traumatic or upsetting memory are addressed through an eight-phase approach which includes history taking, assessment, body scan, etc. [25]. The process and procedures are directed by the adaptive information processing model which reduces the long-term influence of distressing traumatic memory through the adaptive coping mechanisms [25–27].

4.3.4 Play Therapy

Play therapy is a way of expressing incidents and emotions through normal, self-guided, self-healing method among children aged 3–11. Children who are unable to deal directly with trauma and suffer from PTSD are helped through this technique. Games, drawings, and other methods are used to help in the process of traumatic memories of children by the therapists [28].

4.3.5 Group Therapy

Survivors of trauma keenly feel their isolation from the rest of the world. They avoid the connection with other people and place. For this reason group therapy has developed an important place among healing and recovery approaches. The role of the group leader is to facilitate discussion and to manage the relational dynamics in the group. Survivors of related traumatic developments share their experience and responses to them in group therapy. Through discussion group members help each other understand that many people would have done the same thing in the comparable situation.

Topics for trauma groups include education about psychological effect of trauma and its long-term effects, how to combat negative self-images, grounding, self-soothing techniques and lessons about the body, victims' strengths, and other critical subjects [29].

4.3.6 Psychodynamic Psychotherapy

The main focus of this therapy is on helping the individual look at how personal values, behavior, and experiences during the traumatic event affect survivors.

4.3.7 Family Therapy

This therapy is essential in cases of traumatized children. This therapy requires the presence of all family members throughout the therapy process. All family members are affected when any traumatic event occurs, and parents or caretakers have parallel feelings of denial, anger, shock, confusion, helplessness, etc. The loss of self-control, the impulsiveness, and the extreme aversive character of the event(s) are principal pathogenic elements of PTSD. Family and parental support play a vital part in deciding the effect of traumatic incident on child (Shaffer) [30–32].

4.3.8 Specific Parent: Child Therapy

1. Filial therapy
2. Parent-child interaction therapy

Filial therapy: To treat emotional and behavioral difficulties in children, Bernard Gurney in 1964 formulated filial therapy, the first parent-child play therapy to have a play-like approach. Filial therapy [33] is an evidence-based structured approach to restoring and enhancing parent-child relationships. This therapy improves emotional connectedness, communication, and conflict negotiation [33, 34].

Parent-child interaction therapy is another therapy for enhancing parent-child relationship. It was developed by Sheila Eyberg [24]. The aim of this therapy is highly specified which includes separate sessions of each parent/caretakers and then with parents and child together.

There are many treatment modalities to work with survivors. Many researchers are excited to work and give expressive therapy for traumatized children and adolescents. The parent-child relationship along with family dynamics, levels of adaptation, and coping between parents and child is important for child's adjustment in the aftermath of a traumatic incident. Meyer suggested the need for protective, preventive, and educational measures to prevent all types of accidents in children. But unfortunately, awareness about such situations and measures reaches people after the incident has occurred. A door-to-door campaign of awareness and prevention has been suggested that might help to prevent all possible occurrences. Counseling or systematic psychodiagnosis of the child and parents might result in successful total rehabilitation of a child who underwent major trauma like amputation.

In counseling sessions victims are asked to focus and appreciate how they are still alive and recognize what they possess rather than what they have lost. They are encouraged to consider the strength it takes to get as far as they have got and that they deserve a well-earned credit. Spirituality is a way of linking with inner self. Religion, meditation, music, having hope, and dreams can be developed by spirituality. It also helps people understand that physical looks are less important than their overall personality [34, 35].

Conclusion

Trauma significantly affects the children's physical, behavioral, and emotional condition. It has become essential to know how traumas affect children as well as family members and how to help them to cope with psychological hazards. Due to trauma, different psychological disorders developed (e.g., depression, anxiety, PTSD), and it directly affects the child's overall functioning. To manage the child and his family, psychotherapist plays an important role. Using different psychological techniques, therapist makes children and their family to cope with trauma and manage their psychological present status independently. Flexible and integrative approach to treatment is suggested in order to address the multifaceted and changing requirements of individual trauma survivors.

References

1. American Psychiatric Association. Diagnostic and statistical manual of mental disorders. 4th ed. Washington, DC: American Psychiatric Association; 1994.
2. American Psychiatric Association. Diagnostic and statistical manual of mental disorders. 5th ed. Arlington: APA; 2013.
3. Brach T. Mindful presence: a foundation for compassion and wisdom. In: Germer CK, Siegel RD, editors. Wisdom and compassion in psychotherapy: deepening mindfulness in clinical practice. New York: Guildford; 2011. ISBN: 978-1462518869.
4. Baker SP, O'Neil B, Hoddon W, Long WB. The injury severity score: a method for describing patients with multiple injuries and evaluating emergency care. J Trauma. 1974;14(3):187–96.
5. Briere J. Trauma symptom checklist for children: professional manual. Odessa: Psychological Assessment Resources, Inc.; 1996.
6. Bryant RA, Moulds ML, Nixon RV. Cognitive behaviour therapy of acute stress disorder: a four-year follow-up. Behav Res Ther. 2003;41(4):489–94.
7. Holder Y, Peden M, Krug EG, Johan L. World Health Organization. Department of Injuries and Violence Prevention; 2001.
8. Bryant RA, Sackville T, Dang ST, Moulds M, Guthrie R. Treating acute stress disorder: an evaluation of cognitive behavior therapy and supportive counseling techniques. Am J Psychiatr. 1999;152(11):1780–6.
9. Kilpatrick DG, Ruggiero KJ, Acierno R, Saunders BE, Resnick MS, Best CL. Violence and risk of PTSD, major depression, substance abuse/dependency, and co-morbidity: results from the National Survey of Adolescents. J Consult Clin Psychol. 2003;71(4):692–700.
10. Zoladz P. Current status on behavioral and biological markers of PTSD: a search for clarity in a conflicting literature. Neurosci Biobehav Rev. 2013;37(5):860–95.
11. Wyatt GE, Carmona JV, Loeb TB, Ayala A, Chin D. Sexual abuse. In: Wingood GM, DiClemente RJ, editors. Handbook of women's sexual and reproductive health. Issues in women's health. New York: Kluwer Academic/Plenum Publishers; 2002. p. 195–216.
12. Lobel CM. Relationship between childhood sexual abuse and borderline personality disorder in women psychiatric inpatients. J Child Sex Abuse. 1992;1(1):63–80.
13. Ministry of law and justice, Government of India. The gazette of India: the protection of children from sexual offences act, 2012. New Delhi: The Controller of Publication; 2012.
14. Burman MA, Stein JA, Golding JM, Seigel JM, Sorenson SB, Forsythe AB, Tees CA. Sexual assault and mental disorders in a community population. J Consult Clin Psychol. 1988;56(6):843–50.
15. Faulstich ME, Carey MP, Ruggiero L, et al. Assessment of depression in childhood and adolescence: an evaluation of the Center for Epidemiological Studies Depression Scale for Children (CES-DC). Am J Psychiatr. 1986;143(8):1024–7.
16. Brymer M, Layne C, Jacobs A, Pynoos R, Ruzek J, Steinberg A, et al. (National Child Traumatic Stress and National Center for PTSD). Psychological first aid field operations guide. 2nd ed. 2006.
17. Nader KO. Kriegler JA. Blake DD. Clinician administered PTSD scale, Child and Adolescent Version (CAPS-C) White River Junction: National Center for PTSD; 1998.
18. Nader K. Psychometric review of Childhood PTS Reaction Index (CPTS-RI). In: Stamm BH, editor. Measurement of stress, trauma, and adaptation. Lutherville: Sidran Press; 1996. p. 83–6.

19. Nash WP, Watson PJ. Review of VA/DOD clinical practice guideline on management of acute stress and interventions to prevent posttraumatic stress disorder. J Rehabil Res Dev. 2012;49(5):637–48.
20. Saigh P, Yaski AE, Oberfield RA, Green BL, Halamandaris PV, Rubenstein H, Nester J, Resko J, Hetz B, McHugh M. The children's PTSD inventory: development and reliability. J Trauma Stress. 2000;30:369–80.
21. Copes WS, Champion HR, Sacco WJ, Lawnick MM, Keast SL, Bain LW. The injury severity score revised. J Trauma. 1988;28(1):69–77.
22. Trauma ORG. Merck manual. Modified Glasgow coma scale for infants and children. 2008.
23. Eifling K, Moy HP. Evidence-based EMS: disaster scenarios and psychological first aid. 2015.
24. Eyberg S. PCIT: integration of traditional and behavioural concerns. Child Behav Ther. 1988;10:33–46.
25. Hughes M. EMDR as a therapeutic treatment for complex regional pain syndrome: a case report. J EMDR Pr Res. 2014;8(2):66–73.
26. Shapiro F. Efficacy of the eye movement desensitization procedure in the treatment of traumatic memories. J Trauma Stress. 1989;2(2):199–223.
27. Shapiro F, Laliotis D. EMDR and the adaptive information processing model: integrative treatment and case conceptualization. Clin Soc Work J. 2010;39(2):191–200.
28. Flannery RB, Everly GS. Crisis intervention: a review. Int J Emerg Ment Health. 2000;2(2):119–26.
29. Foa B, Keane TM, Friedman MJ, Cohen JA, editors. Effective treatments for PTSD: practice guidelines from the International Society for Traumatic Stress Studies. 2nd ed. New York: Guilford Press; 2009.
30. North CS, Pfefferbaum B. Mental health response to community disasters: a systematic review. JAMA. 2013;310(5):507–18.
31. Nucifora FC Jr, Subbarao I, Hsu EB. Changing the paradigm: a novel framework for the study of resilience. Int J Emerg Ment Health. 2012;14(1):73–6.
32. Shaffer D, Fisher P, Dulcan M, et al. The NIMH Diagnostic Interview Schedule for Children (DISC-2.3): description, acceptability, prevalence and performance in the MECA study. J Am Acad Child Adolesc Psychiatry. 2000;39:28–38.
33. Guerney L. Filial therapy. In: Schaefer CE, editor. Foundations of play therapy. New York: Wiley; 2003. p. 99–142.
34. Rye N. Filial therapy for enhancing relationships in families. J Fam Health Care. 2008;18(5):179–81.
35. Weissman MM, Orvaschel H, Padian N. Children's symptom and social functioning self-report scales: comparison of mothers' and children's reports. J Nerv Ment Dis. 1980;168(12):736–40.

5

Nidhi Sugandhi

5.1 Background

The lack of dedicated national trauma registry in India and other Asian and African countries is the major hurdle in assessment of the exact incidence of paediatric trauma, its causes and its burden on the society in terms of morbidity and mortality. However, studies from few single tertiary care institutions have observed that trauma admissions constitute 10–20% of all paediatric admissions [1, 2], with almost 6–10% of children succumbing to their injuries.

Unfortunately the real number is expected to be much higher as this number would not include children affected in extremes, i.e. minor trauma which is treated by primary health centres or paramedical personnel or those who succumb to major trauma immediately and cannot make it to any health-care facility.

The management of paediatric trauma has unfortunately been ignored, even in Western countries but especially in developing world where it is overshadowed by the quantum of communicable diseases. However, many of the deaths in this category are avoidable if prompt, aggressive and specialized treatment is undertaken, right from the incidence of injury [3, 4].

The management of paediatric trauma is a very intricate process requiring highly trained and dedicated individuals and specialized equipment. Most of the time, the paediatric injuries are ignored in the much larger bulk of adult trauma, especially in cases of mass injuries. Because they are dependent members of the society, much of the resources are siphoned off to treat the working adult population, which has undesirable effects on treatment of injured children.

The health-care professionals involved in the management of children need specialized training streamlined towards management of paediatric population. Children are not just small adults; they have a completely different physiology and

N. Sugandhi
Department of Pediatric Surgery, RML, New Delhi, India

© Springer Nature Singapore Pte Ltd. 2018
R. Ahmad Khan, S. Wahab (eds.), *Blunt Abdominal Trauma in Children*,
https://doi.org/10.1007/978-981-13-0692-1_5

31

requirements which the trauma caregiver needs to be proficient with. In the absence of such dedicated professionals, injured children are under high risk of being mismanaged just by virtue of the treatment given being more appropriate for an adult. The same goes for equipment and drugs available in the trauma centre which need to be specialized for the paediatric population.

Also, in the developing world, the health-care facilities are already overwhelmed with communicable and infectious diseases. In those situations, specialized and prompt attention to trauma patients often suffers. The speedy and focused protocol-based approach to an injured child is all but impossible in a general tertiary care centre. Specialty-specific care including neurosurgical, vascular, cardiac, abdominal, urological, thoracic and orthopaedic expertise is also often not available under a single roof.

All these factors underline the absolute need for specialized paediatric trauma centres where all the specialized expertise, trained staff and appropriate equipment are immediately available at a single centre. This is an essential step to minimize mortality and morbidity in paediatric trauma. This chapter deals with the initial stabilization and management of trauma patients from the site of accident till definitive injury-specific treatment is undertaken.

5.2 Prehospital Response

Paediatric trauma differs from adult trauma in many ways due to multifactorial reasons. The most significant of these is that for the same amount of force children almost invariably sustain more severe injuries. This is due to their smaller mass resulting in greater force per unit weight and also due to unique anatomical and physiological considerations such as more elastic tissue and less bony protection. Due to their smaller physiological reserve, they are also more susceptible to succumb to trauma. Considering these factors, the bottom line remains that for best possible outcomes, the resuscitation and treatment of children with trauma should start right at the site of injury, rather than wait for them to be transported to a health-care facility.

The concept of 'golden hour' was introduced by Crowley in 1979 and refers to the first hour after a traumatic injury, management during which time is most critical for decreasing mortality and optimizing prognosis [5]. This concept of golden hour has stood the test of time, and many studies have validated the effectiveness of early treatment initiation during this time period. In fact, early resuscitation initiated during this period has been found to reduce mortality by 25–30% [5–7].

Trunkey in 1983 described a typical 'trimodal distribution' of deaths in relation to paediatric trauma [8]. Accordingly, most of the deaths in children following trauma occur either immediately (Group 1), within minutes to hours (Group 2) or after days to weeks (Group 3). Group 1 deaths are due to severe trauma resulting in immediate loss of life as, for example, in severe injuries to the brainstem or great vessels. Group 2 constitutes those with mass lesion injuries of the central nervous system and abdominal or thoracic structures, whereas Group 3 constitutes delayed deaths due to sepsis or multiorgan failure. Evidently, Group 2 is where the patients can benefit most in terms of decreased mortality by early prehospital initiation of resuscitation. However it has been shown that early prehospital treatment also decreases mortality in Group 3 by preventing triggering of harmful uncontrolled physiological cascades leading to delayed complications [9].

Thus, the ultimate aim is to get the injured child to a specialized centre as quickly as possible where definitive treatment can be initiated, at the same time, not losing precious initial hours for initiating treatment which can have life and death consequences. To this end, the prehospital response has to be carefully balanced and prioritized between 'treat' and '*scoop and run*', i.e.:

1. Immediate treatment/first aid/resuscitation at the site of the incident
2. Evacuation and transport to a tertiary care centre or specialized trauma centre

Various factors need to be considered while making this decision. The severity and mechanism of injury, age of the child involved, available facilities for first aid/resuscitation, distance to the trauma centre and means of transport available, availability of specialized trauma and transport teams are few of the practical problems that need to be considered.

5.2.1   On-Site Treatment and Resuscitation

Management of trauma requires a structured response as detailed in Table 5.1 [10].

Considering the absolute need of early treatment, the trained transport team needs to initiate at least the first steps including the primary survey and resuscitation at the site of accident. The investigations needed in the primary survey may not always be possible on-site unless the transport ambulance is equipped with

Table 5.1 Structured approach for treatment of an injured child

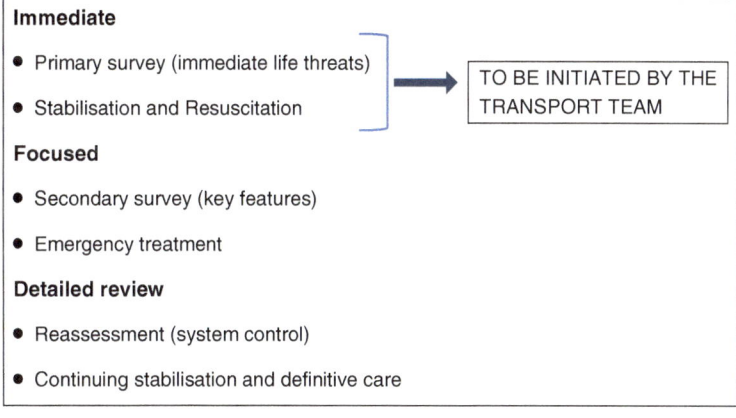

radiographers and X-ray and USG machines. Even so, whatever is possible should be carried out to stabilize, assess and resuscitate the injured child.

5.2.1.1 Primary Survey and Resuscitation by Trained Transport Personnel

Throughout the primary survey, acutely fatal problems are identified and treated simultaneously. This consists of a rapid 'physiological' examination and resuscitation as laid out in Table 5.2 [10].

Though the normal approach to any seriously ill individual follows an 'ABCDE' approach, catastrophic external haemorrhage can quickly exsanguinate and cause death in a small child. Hence, its control takes precedence over everything else. In major trauma <C> ABCDE has become the conventional methodology.

Haemorrhage

Evident severe external bleeding demands the immediate precedence over other features. This needs to be identified on first inspection and controlled by direct pressure, dressings or tourniquet. Tranexamic acid if available should be given in the dose of 15 mg/kg.

Airway and Cervical Spine

The airway and cervical spine need to be assessed simultaneously. Any visible obstruction to the airway should be removed with a finger sweep. Tongue fall is an important and most common cause of airway obstruction in an unconscious patient and can be dealt with an oral Guedel's airway. Active suctioning and oxygen should be started.

Before undertaking advanced airway intervention and for the purpose of transport, the cervical spine needs to be assessed and stabilized; otherwise any minor injury can be worsened by the movement and result in permanent and severe morbidity. Cervical spine injury is presumed in cases of injuries to the face and neck, high impact falls and high-speed vehicular accidents, even if definitive evidence by means of an X-ray is not be available in the field. If definitive exclusion is not possible, cervical spine injury should be presumed to be present and cervical spine immobilization carried out before undertaking advanced interventions on the airway. The cervical spine immobilization needs to be semi-rigid as fixed immobilizations in a struggling or irritable child may exacerbate the injury. Manual in-line immobilization or immobilization using a head block and strapping can secure the cervical spine.

Table 5.2 Primary survey	• C > ABCDE
	• Catastrophic external haemorrhage>
	• Airway (with cervical spine control)
	• Breathing with ventilatory support
	• Circulation with haemorrhage control
	• Disability with prevention of secondary insult
	• Exposure with temperature control

Advanced airway manoeuvres include bag and mask ventilation and endotracheal intubation. These need to be carried out not only in established airway obstruction but also in predicted airway obstruction like in case of inhalational burns. While intubating an injured child, head tilt and chin raise are not advisable as these may worsen the injury to the cervical spine. Intubation should be done only with jaw thrust. Rarely airway may need to be secured surgically, for example, tracheostomy or cricothyroidotomy, but this can only be carried out if a doctor is a part of the transfer team.

The on-field airway management of airway is summarized in Table 5.3.

Breathing

Adequacy of breathing is confirmed by checking the respiratory effort, efficacy and adequacy of oxygen delivery to the other organ systems. This is done in the same way as airway assessment, namely, by 'looking, listening and feeling'. Asymmetrical chest movements, surgical emphysema, tracheal deviation and resonant percussion are dangerous signs which may possibly indicate pneumothorax, hemothorax, flail chest, etc. These are clinical diagnosis, and it is not necessary to wait for any imaging to confirm and treat these conditions. These require immediate intervention in the form of intercostal drainage either with an intercostal tube or needle decompression. This needs to be done on the site of injury itself. Fully trauma-trained nurse and paramedical staff should be able to carry out such interventions; otherwise presence of a doctor becomes necessary. Inadequate respiratory efforts (unconscious patient), failure of breathing mechanism (e.g. flail chest) and constant hypoxia necessitate manual or mechanical ventilation.

Circulation

The assessment of circulation in the primary survey entails the quick estimation of pulse rate, pulse volume, heart rate and rhythm and peripheral perfusion like colour, temperature and capillary return and blood pressure. Table 5.4 lists out indicators of circulatory compromise for which immediate measures need to be initiated.

Table 5.3 On-site airway management

• Look, listen and feel for airway obstruction, respiratory arrest, depression or distress
– Foreign matter in the mouth (blood clot, vomitus, tooth or soil)
– Injury to the structures in the wall (the oral cavity structures, pharyngeal, laryngeal or tracheal injury)
– Pressure from outside, e.g. compression from a prevertebral haematoma in the neck
• Execute essential airway-opening techniques
• Administer high flow oxygen
• Perform suction and cleaning
• Airway supports if necessary
• Intubate if required
• Surgical intubation techniques (e.g. cricothyrotomy)
• Monitoring of oxygen saturation and capnometry in an intubated patient

Table 5.4 Indicators of circulatory compromise requiring intervention

• Increasing heart rate or development of bradycardia
• Decreasing systolic blood pressure
• Peripheral shock (capillary refill time >2 s)
• Tachypnoea unrelated to chest condition
• Altered conscious level without any evidence of head injury

Table 5.5 AVPU score for neurological disability

A—alert
V—responds to voice
P—responds only to pain
U—unresponsive

Vascular access should be established with two large bore intravenous cannulae preferably in the peripheral vein of all the critically injured children. Sometimes central venous cannulation including jugular and femoral veins and even intraosseous access may be necessary.

At presentation if the child is haemodynamically stable, immediate fluid bolus should be avoided. The principle behind this is 'the first clot is the best clot', and extra fluid or blood products in a child not in shock may dislodge the tamponading clot.

If child is assessed to be in shock, immediate volume replacement should be undertaken, initially with crystalloids. It is recommended that colloids be withheld till the source of bleeding is identified and controlled or given only if it is refractory shock not responding to at least three boluses of crystalloids. The trauma team at the centre must be immediately informed to keep blood products ready. If site of haemorrhage is identified, temporary measures such as pressure or tourniquets should be applied. Vasoactive and inotropic drugs may need to be started during transport itself. Cardiac arrest necessitates starting CPR at the site or during transport [11].

Disability

Disability refers to both mental and physical disabilities. Out of these assessment and management of mental disability take immediate precedence. An abbreviated evaluation of the nervous system can establish the consciousness level and basic brain function by assessment of pupil size and reactivity. The AVPU method grades neurological status of the injured as alert, responding to voice, responding to pain or unresponsive (Table 5.5).

Glasgow Coma Score is another scale to assess neurological disability. It has different scoring in infants and older children (Tables 5.6 and 5.7).

Immediate intervention and resuscitation of neurological functions is required in cases where the GCS and AVPU scoring shows that the patient has decompensating head injury. A GCS of less than 8 and/or AVPU score corresponding to 'P' or 'U' requires immediate intervention, and this should be conveyed to the trauma centre/ hospital. The child also needs specialized neurosurgical care and hence should be transferred to a hospital where such expertise is available [12].

Table 5.6 Glasgow Coma Scale for infants and toddlers (4–15 years)

Response		Score
Eye opening	Spontaneously	4
	To verbal stimuli	3
	To pain	2
	No response	1
Best motor response	Obeys verbal command	6
	Localizes to pain	5
	Withdraws to pain	4
	Abnormal flexion to pain (decorticate)	3
	Abnormal extension to pain (decerebrate)	2
	No response	1
Best verbal response	Oriented and converses	5
	Disoriented and converses	4
	Inappropriate words	3
	Incomprehensible sounds	2
	No response to pain	1

Table 5.7 Glasgow Coma Scale for children >4 years

Response		Score
Eye opening	Spontaneously	4
	To verbal stimuli	3
	To pain	2
	No response	1
Best motor response	Spontaneous or obeys verbal command	6
	Localizes to pain or withdraws to touch	5
	Withdraws to pain	4
	Abnormal flexion to pain (decorticate)	3
	Abnormal extension to pain (decerebrate)	2
	No response	1
Best verbal response	Alert, babbles and coos to normal ability	5
	Less than normal words, irritable cry	4
	Cries only to pain	3
	Moans only to pain	2
	No response to pain	1

Exposure and Environment

For proper assessment of a critically injured child, a full exposure by taking off all the clothes is necessary. However, since children become cold very quickly, maintaining a warm environment while examination is important. This can be done by examining in a warm environment inside the ambulance and covering the child with warm blankets. Warm intravenous fluids are also desirable. This also includes avoidance of exposure to any toxic environment.

The imaging and investigations which are normally adjuncts to the primary survey cannot be carried out on-field or during transport and should be planned and done as soon as the child reaches the hospital [13].

5.2.1.2 First Aid by Lay Person/Guardian While Waiting for Medical Help

In developing countries like India, where dedicated trauma transfer teams and trained personnel are not available, such extensive and focused prehospital response is not possible by the lay persons. Neither is the specialized equipment needed is present at the site of injury. Despite this, there are few basic first aid and stabilization measures which the public can be made aware of. These can considerably help in decreasing the immediate mortality and preventing further damage in an injured child.

The first and foremost step is to call and arrange for help followed by attending to the injured child.

A secure airway is the first priority. In the absence of airways and ET tubes, the airway of the child can be cleared by finger sweep method by any lay person and any foreign body or debris removed. To ensure that the secretions or bleeding does not occlude the airway, the head should be tilted back slightly and child placed in a lateral recovery position, i.e. the child should be stabilized laterally so as to allow patent airway and free drainage contents from the oral cavity. The head should be tilted back slightly to ensure an open airway, and the upper hip and knee should be flexed at right angles. Back should be straight and supported. This position ensures that the airway is not obstructed by tongue fall in an unconscious child and all the secretions including any internal bleeding drain outside rather than compromise the airway.

Transport of the child should be done on a rigid board (e.g. a wooden plank) which ensures minimum movement of the spine rather than on a loose cloth or holding by all limbs which can seriously damage the spinal cord in an injured spine. Commonly available any rigid object can be used as splints for stabilization such as pillows, paper rolls, etc. Simple injury-specific interventions include measures like thorough washing of burn wounds, splinting of fractured limbs, etc.

Normothermia can be maintained even in cold seasons by simply covering up the child in warm blankets.

Visible severe external haemorrhage can be limited by direct pressure or dressings fashioned out of common household items like clean cloth. Indigenous materials like cloth or elastic materials may be used as temporary tourniquet.

Someone trained in first aid can even initiate CPR at the simplest recommendation of 30 compressions for two ventilations.

5.2.2 Evacuation and Transport of an Injured Child

In case no local treatment or management facilities are available, then transfer of the injured victim to specialized centre becomes the priority. This is covered in detail in Sect. 5.2.

5.3 Evacuation and Transport of an Injured Child

The goal of a transport team is to transfer the child to a specialized facility in the quickest possible time, while initiating stabilization and resuscitative measures simultaneously. The transfer can be undertaken by road, air or other means depending on the local conditions. Air transport offers advantage in speed, avoidance of traffic and regionalization of specialized care but is not possible in all countries due to monetary and geographical considerations. Such emergency medical service is highly advanced in the USA, Australia, Germany, etc. where it was developed based on models of emergency units in service in Korea and Vietnam wars [1, 2].

A trained trauma team and a PALS compliant transport ambulance are a prerequisite for such transfers. The transport vehicle should have all the basic resuscitative equipment in all sizes required for children. The suggested equipment that is needed is stated in Table 5.8. It is not necessary for a physician to always be present on the transfer team, but trained nurses and paramedical staff capable of obtaining at least basic airway, intravenous access, care of spine, etc. are absolutely mandatory. Various studies have been conducted into the constitution of the trauma team and recommendations put forward. The suggested constitution of a trauma transfer team is elucidated in Table 5.9. This can be modified according to the local conditions and availability. In fact, according to some studies, the need for a physician to be present in the transfer team can be accurately assessed on a case-to-case basis depending on the history available.

When summoned to a site of accident or injury, time is of utmost importance. The transfer team needs to carry out a quick assessment of the injury and its severity. This information is not only important for deciding how to immobilize and transport an injured child but also to start early resuscitation measures during transport itself. In addition, this information needs to be relayed to the team leader of the trauma centre where the child is being transferred. The basic information that needs

Table 5.8 Suggested list of equipment necessary in a transport ambulance	1. Endotracheal tubes—all sizes and intubation equipment including laryngoscopes
	2. Airways—all sizes
	3. Warmed intravenous fluids
	4. Intravenous access cannulas, intraosseous cannulas, arterial lines and central venous lines
	5. Nasogastric tubes—all sizes
	6. Foley's catheter—all sizes
	7. Blood pressure cuffs
	8. Cervical collars and spine stabilization boards
	9. Inotropes and resuscitative drugs
	10. Suction and oxygen supply
	11. Monitoring equipment
	12. USG Doppler if possible
	13. Radio and communication equipment

Table 5.9 Suggested manpower for a trauma transfer team

1. Nurse trained in trauma and PALS
2. Paramedical staff trained in trauma and PALS
3. Driver
4. Radiographer if possible
5. Paediatric physician or intensivist if need assessed

Table 5.10 Preliminary information and assessment of the injured child for transport and reception preparedness—ATMISTER

A Age/sex/weight
T Time of incident
M Mechanism of injury
I Injury suspected
S Signs including vital signs, Glasgow Coma Scale
T Treatment so far
E Estimated time of arrival to emergency department
R Requirements, i.e. bloods, specialist services, tiered response, ambulance call

to be assimilated and conveyed to the trauma centre is lined out in Table 5.10 [10]. The communication needs to be dynamic, especially in long transfers, i.e. any change in status during transfer should be transmitted immediately to the trauma centre so that adequate modifications can be made.

References

1. Ford EG, Andrassy RJ, editors. Pediatric trauma- initial assessment and management. Philadelphia: WB Saunders Company; 1994.
2. DeRoss A, Vane DW. Early evaluation and resuscitation of the pediatric trauma patient. Semin Pediatr Surg. 2004;13(2):74–9.
3. Sharma M, Lahoti BK, Khandelwal G, Mathur RK, Sharma SS, Laddha A. Epidemiological trends of pediatric trauma: a single-center study of 791 patients. J Indian Assoc Pediatr Surg. 2011;16(3):88–92.
4. Tandon JN, Kalra A, Kalra K, Sahu SC, Nigam CB, Qureshi GU. Profile of accidents in children. Indian Pediatr. 1993;30:765–9.
5. Crowley RS. Foreword. Am Surg. 1979;45:77–8.
6. Border JR, Lewis FR, Aprahamin C, et al. Panel: Prehospital trauma care- stabilize or scoop and run. J Trauma. 1983;23:708–11.
7. Ramenofsky ML, Luterman A, Curreri PW, et al. EMS for paediatrics: optimum treatment or unnecessary delay? J Pediatr Surg. 1983;18:498–504.
8. Trunkey DD. Trauma. Sci Am. 1983;249:28–35.
9. Stafford PW, Blinman TA, Nance ML. Practical points in evaluation and resuscitation of the injured child. Surg Clin North Am. 2002;82:273–301.
10. Samuels M, Wieteska S, editors. Advanced paediatric life support: a practical approach to emergencies. 6th ed. Hoboken: Wiley; 2016.
11. Tepas JJ, Mollitt DL, Talbert JF, et al. The pediatric trauma score as a predictor of injury severity in the injured child. J Paediatr Surg. 1987;22:14–8.
12. PAM R, AAF A, editors. Surgical emergencies in children – a practical guide. Oxford: Butterworth Heinemann Ltd.; 1994.
13. Center for Disease control and Prevention. Guidelines for field triage of injured patients. Morbidity and Mortality Weekly Report. 2009;58.

Assessment of a Child with Abdominal Trauma

6

Rizwan Ahmad Khan

Trauma involving the abdomen is the most common cause of death in children due to unrecognized injury. In pediatric emergency, a significant portion of workload on a pediatric surgeon is to assess an injured child with blunt abdominal trauma. Pediatric trauma differs from adult trauma in many ways, e.g., mechanisms, injury patterns, anatomy, and long-term effects on growth and development. A focused clinical examination diagnoses most of the important injuries and avoids unnecessary management delays and investigations. Diagnosing intra-abdominal injury is the crux of the examination. Intra-abdominal organs can be injured either by blunt or penetrating injuries. Blunt injuries are much more common than penetrating injuries (85% vs 15%). Pediatric internal organs are more likely to be injured owing to a smaller torso, larger and more mobile viscera, and decreased amount of intra-abdominal fat [1, 2].

The smaller body size leads to greater distribution of injury to other body parts rather than restricted to the impact site. Therefore, it is pertinent to be very thorough in examining an injured child [3].

6.1 Systemic Assessment and Stabilization

The core principles of the Advanced Trauma Life Support algorithm apply to preliminary treatment of abdominal trauma is similar in the pediatric as well [2].

R. A. Khan
Department of Pediatric Surgery, Jawaharlal Nehru Medical College, AMU, Aligarh, India

© Springer Nature Singapore Pte Ltd. 2018
R. Ahmad Khan, S. Wahab (eds.), *Blunt Abdominal Trauma in Children*,
https://doi.org/10.1007/978-981-13-0692-1_6

6.1.1 Primary Survey and Resuscitation

The aim of the primary survey is to identify immediately fatal injuries. These conditions must be managed as they are diagnosed with ongoing primary survey. It includes:

1. Airway management and cervical spine protection (Fig. 6.1):
   (a) A patient with a suspected cervical spine injury (e.g., neck pain, neurological deficit, unconscious, or suggestive mode of trauma) must be immobilized with the neck in a neutral position to prevent further spinal injury. The patient should be restricted on a spine board, and closely fitting hard cervical collar should be applied. The other indicators of cervical spine injury are first rib fracture, associated with abdominal and thoracic injury. The patients' airway should always be unobstructed. Noisy or labored respiration or paradoxical movements of the chest are signs of airway obstruction. The oral cavity must be cleansed of any vomitus, blood, or other foreign materials manually or with a suction catheter. The airway obstruction due to falling tongue may be secured by a plain chin lift and/or jaw thrust. It may also necessitate advanced airway management techniques. When utilized, an oropharyngeal or the nasopharyngeal airway must be of correct size and inserted properly. The airway is assessed by asking the verbal patients questions or assessing for phonation in nonverbal patients. Consideration must be given to immediate intubation if there is difficulty in bag–valve–mask ventilation, <8 score on Glasgow Coma Scale, hypoxemia, hypoventilation, decompensated shock patient not responsive to fluid resuscitation, or loss of protective airway reflexes. Intubation of a child requires consideration of age, size, and mechanism of injury. In general, cuffed endotracheal tubes are safe in infants and young children. However, uncuffed tubes are generally used in children <8 years old unless there is a need for a cuffed tube. For children ages 1–10 years, the following formulas estimate the proper size of endotracheal tube: uncuffed endotracheal tube size (internal diameter) 5 (age in years 1 16)/4 and cuffed endotracheal tube size (internal diameter) 5 (age in years 1 12)/4 [3, 4].
   (b) Whenever required, intravenous anesthesia (rapid sequence induction) should only be used by a skilled anesthesiologist when successful intubation of the trachea with patients cervical spine being immobilized cervical spine can be guaranteed. In cases of severe facial trauma, cricothyrotomy should be performed.
2. Breathing:
   (a) High flow oxygen must be given to every patient. Any difficulty in breathing must be noticed by carefully inspecting for tracheal deviation or asymmetrical chest expansion. Pulse oximetry and capnography must be employed to monitor adequate perfusion and arterial oxygen saturation as well as to confirm endotracheal tube position [5].

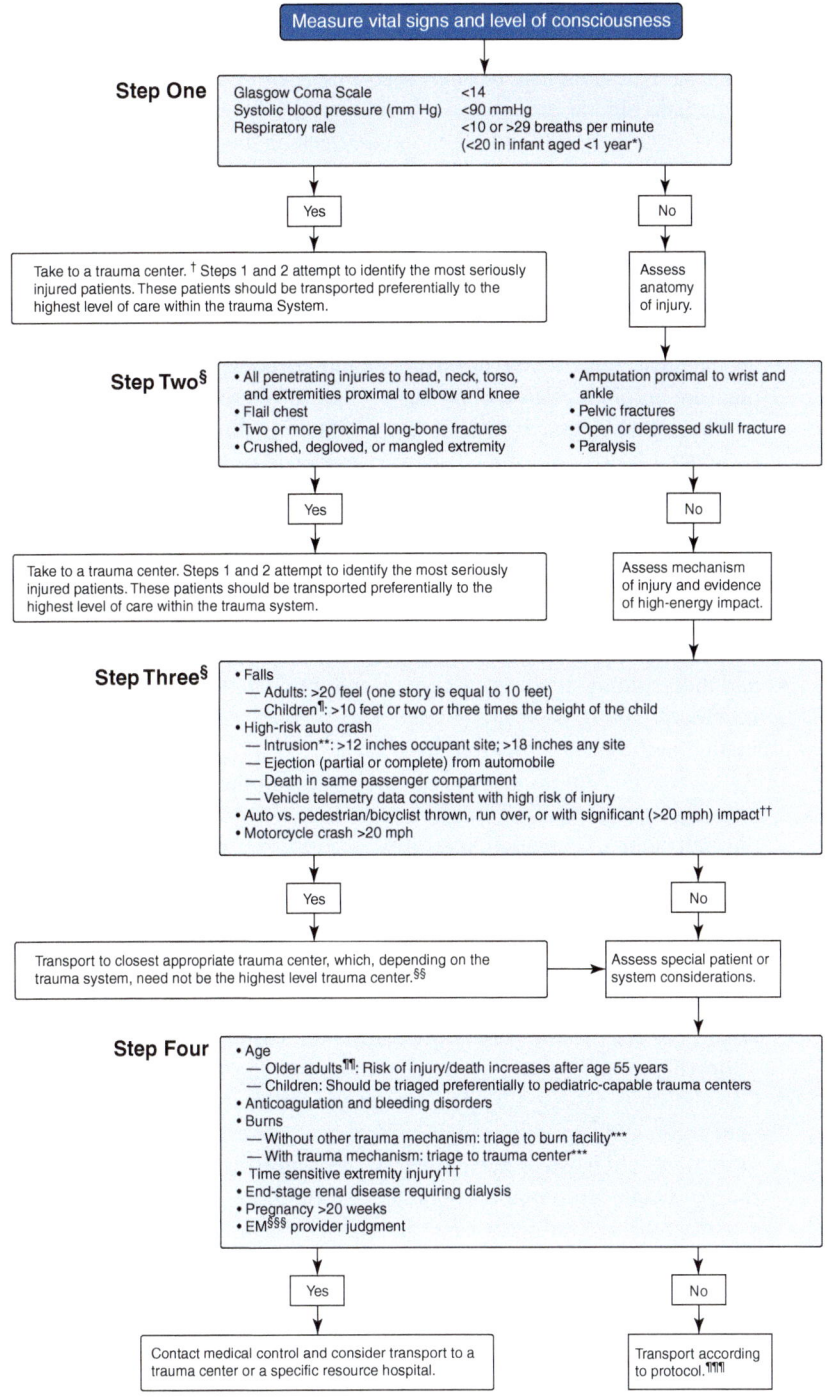

Fig. 6.1 CDC protocol for tiered response to pediatric trauma triage in the USA

(b) The respiratory conditions which need instantaneous handling are massive hemothorax, tension pneumothorax, and flail chest.

A massive hemothorax is often associated with cardiovascular instability. Immediate pleural drainage is required, and if the initial volume of blood loss is more than 1500 mL or blood drainage is more than 200 mL/h, a thoracotomy should be planned immediately.

If tension pneumothorax is suspected, a wide bore needle should be placed in the thoracic cavity at the level of second intercostal space in the mid-clavicular line. This is followed by proper intercostal tube drainage connected to underwater seal drain. Positive pressure ventilation may lead to conversion of a simple pneumothorax to tension pneumothorax. Therefore an intercostal chest tube drainage should be considered as a prophylactic measure before initiation of positive pressure ventilation.

Flail chest segment leads to considerable hypoxia depending upon the associated lung contusion. If there is evidence of deteriorating respiratory failure despite high flow oxygen and satisfactory pain control (epidural or intercostal blocks), then consideration should be given to immediate intubation and positive pressure ventilation.

(c) The presence of massive surgical emphysema and X-ray showing pneumomediastinum and pneumopericardium points to disruption in major branch of the tracheobronchial tree. These patients need immediate endotracheal and thoracotomy. In these cases even endobronchial intubation may become necessary.

3. Circulation and control of hemorrhage [6]:

(a) As soon as the venous access is established, volume resuscitation must start with appropriate fluid. This should be followed by blood transfusion and normalization of coagulation profile.

(b) Continued hypotension in an abdominal trauma patient warrants search for cardiogenic failure. These patients may have associated cardiac injury, either myocardial contusion (blunt trauma) or cardiac tamponade (penetrating chest injury) leading to rise in jugular venous pressures, muffling of heart sounds, hypotension, increasing tachycardia, and pulsus paradoxus. In these children urgent needle pericardiocentesis for cardiac tamponade can be life-saving [7].

(c) Circulation is assessed by physical examination findings including pulse, skin color, and capillary refill. Children have an extraordinary capacity for vasoconstriction, so a normal blood pressure does not rule out hemorrhagic shock. Minimum acceptable systolic blood pressures based on age are 60 mm Hg in term neonates (0–28 days), 70 mmHg in infants (1–12 months), 70 mm Hg x (2 - age in years) in children between 1 to 10 years of age, and 90 mmHg in children 10 years of age or older. In a hypovolemic patient, a bolus infusion of 20 mL/kg of isotonic crystalloid should be initiated promptly. In a patient with obvious hemorrhage, the use of blood products is advocated as the initial resuscitative measure with prompt surgical control of bleeding.

4. Disorders of the central nervous system:

The central nervous system must be rapidly evaluated by gauging the level of consciousness of the child, spinal cord reflexes, and reaction of pupils to light. The consciousness level is determined by recording the patient's eye opening response and motor response to different stimuli (unprompted, following direct questioning, in response to pain or no response). The spinal cord function is assessed by performing sensory reflexes in all four limbs.

5. Exposure of the whole body:

All children with polytrauma injuries must be fully undressed to permit a comprehensive inspection for detecting injuries. The clothes may be cut off to avoid unnecessary movement of the child with suspected spine injury. However, consideration must also be given to the labile temperature control in the injured child. Therefore the examination room must be kept warm to prevent hypothermia [6].

6.1.2 Secondary Survey

After the primary survey and resuscitation, the patient must undergo a systematic secondary survey with the aim to identify any traumatic injuries not identified on primary survey along with a more detailed history. A head-to-toe inspection is performed, focusing on pupillary size and reactivity; palpation of cranium and cervical spine; palpation of the mid-face for stability; palpation of the chest and abdomen for crepitus or tenderness; inspection of each extremity for deformity, strength, and sensation; inspection and palpation of the cervical, thoracic, and lumbar spine for tenderness or deformity; and examination of the perineum for injury or open fracture often with a rectal examination for sphincter tone. An AMPLE history may be taken, which includes allergies, medications, past medical history, last meal, and events and details explaining the injury. During the course of secondary survey, the essentials of the primary survey, i.e., airway, breathing, and circulation, must also be regularly reassessed.

Tetanus immunization and broad-spectrum antibiotics can be given at this stage. An appropriate history and trauma X-ray series, lateral cervical spinal view, thoracic X-ray, and pelvic view must be obtained. A top-to-toe examination must be done with special emphasis on abdominal examination [7–9].

6.1.3 Tertiary Survey

This in an ongoing process for assessment for minor or missed injuries. This is usually performed about 24 h after arrival—"after the dust settles," this again is a continuing process until the patient is discharged [9].

6.2   Triage and Tiered Response

The process of stratifying and prioritizing treatment according to the severity is triage. This concept originated during the World Wars when the number of inured soldiers far exceeded the capacity of medical attention available and treatment had to be arranged to save maximum lives. In cases of mass casualties or disasters, where resources are limited and the injured victims far exceed the capacity of treatment, the management of the victims needs to be prioritized according to the severity of injury and their salvageability. This ensures that the most serious patients requiring immediate attention and intervention are identified immediately and offered prompt treatment, thus saving maximum lives while ensuring optimum resource utilization. Triage also helps in prognosticating the outcomes in injured victims [3, 4].

During the process of triage, all victims are quickly assessed and assigned a particular priority level, usually ranging from one to five. The type and promptness of response is decided by the risk or triage category that the patient is put into. These levels are usually color coded for ease of identification. Table 6.1 elucidates the color-coded scale usually used to triage patients in the USA, Canada, and Australia. The name, color, and expected response time may vary in different countries, but the concept remains the same (Table 6.1).

It should be remembered that triage is a dynamic process and the injured needs to be reassessed periodically. The priority level can move up or down the scale depending on the changing condition of the child, and the team needs to respond accordingly.

6.2.1   Criteria for Pediatric Trauma Triage

Evidently, objective criteria need to be followed to decide the category and level of attention that a patient needs. Various trauma scoring systems are in use for assessing the severity of injuries the patients. These are based on either anatomical or physiological criteria or both. The simplest among the various scores available is the GCS, and the most commonly used is the Pediatric Trauma Score which uses a combination of physiological and anatomical criteria.

Table 6.1 Triage categories and target times for attending the injured patient [6]

Number	Color	Priority level	Response time to clinician
1	Red	Immediate	0
2	Orange	Very urgent	10
3	Yellow	Urgent	60
4	Green	Standard	240
5	Blue	Nonurgent	None

6.2.1.1 Glasgow Coma Scale

This is the simplest score which categorizes the injured according to their neurological disability. A GCS score of less than eight indicates immediate transfer to a center with specialized neurosurgical care, need for advanced airway management, and an overall poorer prognosis.

6.2.1.2 Pediatric Trauma Score

Introduced by Tepas et al. in 1987, this score is the most popular one in use today and which has the best correlation with severity and outcome [11]. Table 6.2 describes the PTS. The score ranges from −6 to 12. A score of >8 ensures 0% mortality, while a score of 0 correlates with 100% mortality. Also a score of <8 mandates transfer of the patient to specialized pediatric trauma center.

However nowadays a new triage system is recommended which is listed in Table 6.3.

6.2.2 Type of Response

Triage is carried out so that response can be tiered according to the severity of injury. The type of response designated for a particular category depends on the local conditions. For most countries, a GCS or PTS < 8 mandates securing the airway and transfer to a pediatric trauma center with specialized neurosurgery expertise available.

Also, the information regarding transfer of such a child needs to be conveyed to the trauma center in advance so that the whole trauma team is ready with required equipment. Resuscitation of such a child becomes top priority. Trauma specialists with required expertise should already be summoned and kept ready for examination, expert advice, and intervention. Operation theaters, blood and blood products, and intensive care beds should be arranged beforehand.

Every country needs to come up with its own protocol regarding the tiered response to trauma. India still does not have such an organized protocol, especially toward pediatric trauma. An example of how triage can guide the response to pediatric trauma is demonstrated in Fig. 6.1 which gives the CDC guidelines for the trauma patients from the USA [13].

Table 6.2 Pediatric trauma score

	2	1	−1
Size (kg)	>20	10–20	<10
Systolic BP	>90	50–90	<50
Airway	Normal	Secure	Tenous
CNS	Awake	Obtunded	Coma
Open wounds	None	Minor	Major
Fractures	None	Closed	Open

Table 6.3 New triage system

Level A	
Physiology/anatomy/injury	
Airway/breathing	Respiratory compromise or obstruction
	Intubation in the field/ED
	Maxillofacial injuries compromising airway
Circulation	Age-specific hypotension at any time
	<2 years old <60 mmHg
	3–5 years old <70 mmHg
	6–8 years old <80 mmHg
	> 8 years old <90 mmHg
Central nervous system	GCS ≤ 8 with mechanism attributable to trauma
Mechanism	
Penetrating wound	Gross wound to the head, cervical, thoracic, abdomen, or limbs proximal to the elbow/knee (T-shirt and boxer short distribution)—excluding BB wounds
	Penetrating neck or chest wounds
Extremities/skeletal	Amputation of limbs proximal to wrist or ankle
Burns	≥40% TBSA second and third degree combined
	High-voltage electrical injury >600 V
Other	ED attending's discretion in discussion with trauma attending
Level B	
Physiology/anatomy/injury	
Circulation	Uncontrolled hemorrhage
Central nervous system, head, and spine	GCS 9–12
	Head or spine injury with focal neurologic deficit
	Open skull fracture
	Paralysis
Chest	Chest wall deformity
Abdomen	Crush injury
	Pregnancy: 24 weeks by U/S or fundus at umbilicus + abdominal pain/vaginal bleeding from trauma
Extremities/skeletal	2 or more humerus or femur fractures
	Unstable pelvis
	Extremity trauma with neurovascular deficit
Burns	Singed facial or nasal hair
	Burn in enclosed space and suspected inhalation injury
	Burn ≥20% TBSA
Mechanisms (occult injury)	
Penetrating wound (non-GSW)	Head, abdomen, pelvis, groin (T-shirt, boxer short distribution)
Fall	Fall >15 feet
MVC	Ejection from automobile
Level C	
Anatomy	
Central nervous system	GCS 13–14

Table 6.3 (continued)

Neck/chest/abdomen	Seat belt marks with no other level A or B criteria
	Blunt injury with chest, abdomen, or pelvic pain or tenderness
Mechanisms (occult injury)	
MVC	High-risk crash
	Invasion into passenger area with >12 inches at the patient site or >18 inches to any site including roof
	Mortality in the passenger compartment
Motor vehicle versus pedestrian/bicyclist	Thrown or run over
	>20 mph impact
Motorcycle/ATV crash	>20 mph
Burns	$\geq$10 TBSA second and third degree
	<10% TBSA but with circumferential burns
	>1% TBSA to the face, hands, feet, or perineum

6.3   Clinical Assessment of Abdomen

A systematic and skilled approach is needed for proper assessment and evaluation of injuries. A detailed history is necessary to reach to a conclusive clinical diagnosis. The mechanism of injury should be asked, whether there was high velocity transfer (motor vehicle accident) or low velocity (fall or fight) transfer, and site of impact must be ascertained. Enquiry should be made about vomiting and the content (blood, bile). Meticulous and serial physical examination forms the basis of prompt diagnosis and deciding further course of management. Injuries sustained depend on many factors including the size of object, position of the victim, and the way of impact. Neurological impairment suggests evaluation for head injury first, and the patient may be immediately taken up for head CT scan. If the patient is neurologically intact, a methodical physical examination yields valuable information. Inspection of the abdomen may reveal visible abrasions or ecchymoses over the site of impact. Look for any distension. Abdominal pain and tenderness of varying degree may be present. Localized tenderness is associated with minor and diffuse tenderness with major injuries. Signs and symptoms of generalized peritonitis (abdominal rigidity, rebound tenderness, and absent bowel sounds) if firmly established may require an urgent laparotomy without any additional imaging study [8–10]. The patients aged >2 years can be enquired about the presence/absence of abdominal pain and the degree of pain, as mild (pain score 1–3), moderate (pain score 4–6), or severe (pain score 7–10), using the pain scale in place at each institution. The location of abdominal pain was categorized as diffuse, localized, or unknown. The presence, location, and degree of abdominal tenderness on physical examination can be quantified as mild (1–3), moderate (4–6), or severe (7–10) or unknown severity. The location of abdominal tenderness should be categorized as diffuse, above the umbilicus, below the umbilicus, periumbilical, or unknown. The patients should be looked for peritoneal irritation, which can be defined as rebound cough tenderness and guarding. A child with guarding must be treated as potentially unstable, even if he appears clinically stable [11].

In addition, proper auscultation of the abdomen should be performed for detecting the presence or absence of bowel sounds. Finally, results of the rectal examination, if performed, must be documented. A rectal examination should be categorized as positive for blood if gross blood or if the stool is hemoccult-positive. The prostate examination must also be documented (whether high riding or not) [12]. The genital examination is important part of abdominal examination. Enquire about the last void and for any evidence of blood or difficulty in voiding. On examination, look for blood at meatus and scrotal ecchymoses [13].

Any wound should be properly inspected and measured and documentation done. The stab or puncture wounds must be covered with saline-soaked sterile dressings. Moisten the dressing with sterile saline if internal organs are exposed. If there is impalement injury, the impaled object should be stabilized with dressing, and no attempt should be made to remove it.

6.4   Adjunct to Clinical Assessment

Diagnostic peritoneal lavage involves placement of a catheter into the peritoneal cavity, aspiration of free fluid, instillation of normal saline and aspiration of the lavage fluid. Diagnostic peritoneal lavage (DPL) was once a mainstay of trauma evaluations. DPL is very sensitive for detecting hemorrhage and is simple to perform; however it is rarely performed in children as it cannot differentiate inconsequential from significant bleeding, the site, and the grade of injury which are key factors in deciding nonsurgical management of injuries. Since it is an invasive test and is largely replaced by newer assessment tests such as FAST or CT scanning which are faster, noninvasive, and more reliable, the role of DPL is limited to an unstable patient who cannot undergo CT imaging. It may also be used for occult bowel injury where abdominal-free fluid is positive for intestinal contents. DPL may be considered in a patient undergoing emergent decompressive craniotomy (for impending herniation and therefore poor GCS leading to inadequate assessment of the abdomen).

Diagnostic laparoscopy is an excellent tool for further investigation in the hemodynamically stable patient. It can readily localize injury and reduce the rate of negative laparotomy. It a very helpful tool for evaluation in suspected diaphragmatic injuries and suspected bowel injury. In the hands of experienced laparoscopic surgeons, it can be used to manage the repair of injuries including the diaphragm, pancreas, small bowel, and colon.

Diagnostic cystoscopy is another adjunct that can be extremely useful. It can be used to diagnose bladder injuries as well as treat any ureteral injury with stent placement. Evaluation of the ureters is best accomplished with intravenous contrast CT scan with delayed imaging. Suspected injuries can be further evaluated using retrograde fluoroscopic imaging at time of cystoscopy in both blunt and penetrating trauma [5].

References

1. Eppich WJ, Zonfrillo MR. Emergency department evaluation and management of blunt abdominal trauma in children. Curr Opin Pediatr. 2007;19:265–9.
2. Ford EG, Andrassy RJ, editors. Pediatric trauma- initial assessment and management. Philadelphia: WB Saunders Company; 1994.
3. Nakayama DK, Gardner MJ, Rowe MI. Emergency endotracheal intubation in pediatric trauma. Ann Surg. 1900;211:218–23.
4. DeRoss A, Vane DW. Early evaluation and resuscitation of the pediatric trauma patient. Semin Pediatr Surg. 2004;13(2):74–9.
5. Stafford PW, Blinman TA, Nance ML. Practical points in evaluation and resuscitation of the injured child. Surg Clin North Am. 2002;82:273–301.
6. Samuels M, Wieteska S, editors. Advanced paediatric life support: a practical approach to emergencies. 6th ed. Hoboken: Wiley; 2016.
7. Wood J, Rubin DM, Nance ML, et al. Distinguishing inflicted versus accidental abdominal injuries in young children. J Trauma. 2005;59(5):1203–8.
8. Holmes JF, Sokolove PE, Brant WE, Palchak MJ, Vance CW, Owings JT, et al. Identification of children with intra-abdominal injuries after blunt trauma. Ann Emerg Med. 2002;39:500–9.
9. Shlamovitz GZ, Mower WR, Bergman J, Crisp J, DeVore HK, Hardy D, et al. Lack of evidence to support routine digital rectal examination in pediatric trauma patients. Pediatr Emerg Care. 2007;23:537–43.
10. Moss RL, Musemeche CA. Clinical judgment is superior to diagnostic tests in the management of pediatric small bowel injury. J Pediatr Surg. 1996;31:178–82.
11. Jerby BL, Attorri RJ, Morton D. Blunt intestinal injury in children: the role of the physical examination. J Pediatr Surg. 1997;32:580–4.
12. Holmes JF, Nguyen H, Wisner DH. Reliability of the abdominal examination in blunt trauma patients with minor head injury. Acad Emerg Med. 2004;11:513.
13. Taylor GA, O'Donnell R, Sivit CJ. Abdominal injury score: a clinical score for the assignment of risk in children after blunt trauma. Radiology. 1994;190:689–94.

Shagufta Wahab

The decision to advise imaging of the child with suspected intra-abdominal injury begins with clinical evaluation. Since imaging forms the basis of ensuing clinical management including the type of clinical care and monitoring, length of hospital stay, and restriction of activities and follow-up, it takes the center stage in the complete assessment and workup of children following abdominal trauma.

The development of "new" imaging modalities has resulted in a tendency toward giving more importance to newer techniques over the conventional imaging modalities. But conventional methods have their own importance and cannot be replaced [1].

Although the type of injury and the clinical stability of the patient determines the exigency, aptness, and extent of subsequent imaging modalities, plain radiographs of the chest provide a good starting point for initial assessment [1, 2].

7.1 Plain Radiography

Plain X-ray examination is the most common initial imaging that is advised unless the child is hemodynamically unstable. A chest X-ray posteroanterior view and a complete abdominal series are advised if abdominal injury is suspected. Depending on the injury, skeletal imaging of the spine and pelvis is also advised.

Plain radiography may give clues to free fluid in the peritoneal cavity, but they are often subtle. Classic X-ray findings indicating free fluid in peritoneum are bulging of the flanks and central displacement of the bowel loops. The other signs of intraperitoneal fluid collections which can be discerned on careful examination are blurring or indistinct appearance of the inferior angle of the liver and medial displacement of the colon away from the flank and sides. Pneumoperitoneum

S. Wahab
Department of Radiodiagnosis, Jawaharlal Nehru Medical College, AMU, Aligarh, India

© Springer Nature Singapore Pte Ltd. 2018
R. Ahmad Khan, S. Wahab (eds.), *Blunt Abdominal Trauma in Children*,
https://doi.org/10.1007/978-981-13-0692-1_7

indicating gastrointestinal perforation can usually be detected on conventional radiographic studies. However to determine the site of perforation, a gastrointestinal series with water-soluble contrast material needs to be performed. This is indicated if there is any doubt on the origin of pneumoperitoneum or if the operating surgeon wants to know the exact site before laparotomy. They can be localized by performing gastrointestinal contrast study. The gastrointestinal perforations occur in motor vehicle accidents, bicycle handle bar injury or child abuse. Besides duodenal perforation, there can be duodenal wall hematoma. This occurs when duodenum is either compressed against the vertebral column or sheared, resulting in tearing of the submucosal and subserosal vessels within the duodenal wall. Depending upon the size of the hematoma, it can either partly or completely obstruct the duodenum, the bile duct, or the duct of the pancreas. Plain radiographic findings may suggest partial or complete obstruction of the duodenum, usually in the second or third portion. Rarely, the hematoma may appear as a mass, especially if it involves the jejunum or mesentery. An upper GI series can provide a definite diagnosis. Another classic X-ray finding is coil spring mucosal appearance.

Traumatic pancreatitis may lead to findings on plain abdominal radiographs. These include localized ileus due to dilated duodenum and the colon (known as colon cutoff sign). There may be free intraperitoneal fluid and pleural effusion.

Plain radiographic examination in other solid organ injury like hepatic injury is restricted to the detection of gross variations in the size or contour of the liver outline and the detection of free intraperitoneal fluid. Splenic injury is suggested by rib fractures, pneumothorax, significantly elevated or upward shifted left hemidiaphragm, enlargement of the spleen shadow, and signs of free intraperitoneal fluid [1–3].

7.2   Scintigraphy

This is a radionuclide imaging technique in which patients are injected intravenously with a technetium sulfur colloid. This has an affinity to the liver and spleen. After injection of the colloid, scanning is performed on a portable gamma camera with a low-energy, general-purpose collimator. Images are obtained in eight standard directions. Various authors have reported liver spleen scintigraphy almost as "accurate" as is CT. It has been variously reported that scintigraphy is easier to perform than CT, is not affected by motion artefacts, can be easily performed in uncooperative patients also, does not require much sedation, and does not require intravenous or oral contrast administration. Therefore it is supposed to be helpful in evaluating the patient with both head and abdominal injuries and for follow-up. However, it is falsely negative in small lesions; thin, linear lacerations; and injuries to the left lobe of the liver. It takes longer time than abdominal CT, and the absorbed radiation dose to the organs of interest is greater than with CT but not to adjacent organs as happens in CT.

Since scintigraphy is organ-specific, additional imaging is required to assess the adjacent organs [4, 5].

7.3   Excretory Urography

Before the widespread availability of CT scan, excretory urography with nephrography was used to assess the renal integrity and function following abdominal trauma. Nowadays it may be useful for short and quick bedside assessment in an unstable child who is being planned for urgent operative procedure and in patients having minor renal injury presenting as microscopic hematuria. It may be helpful in minor ureteral and bladder leak following abdominal injury. This imaging is also very organ-specific and does not give any information about other retroperitoneal and abdominal structures [2].

7.4   Angiography

Angiography can demonstrate precise bleeding sites and can provide the opportunity for therapeutic intervention (e.g., embolization or pharmacoangiography). However its use for diagnosis of abdominal trauma has become limited with the advent of CT scanning. There are many disadvantages as well like increased cost, loss of diagnostic time, and morbidity due to major complications. Also it does not demonstrate the full extent of injury as well as CT [6].

7.5   Sonography

Sonographic examination is nowadays the primary investigation for assessment of injuries related to blunt nature of abdominal trauma. It is a valuable tool in detecting injury to solid organs both intraperitoneal and retroperitoneal. The ultrasound can detect the presence of free intraperitoneal fluid or blood with good sensitivity. Nowadays with widespread availability of portable ultrasound machines, the trainees or trauma residents need to perform the ultrasound bedside as an adjunct to their clinical assessment. Ultrasound is rapid, inexpensive, noninvasive, and free from radiation and fairly accurate imaging modality for abdominal trauma. However first normal ultrasound examination cannot rule out all kinds of intra-abdominal injury; the reliability and accuracy can be improved by repetitive examinations. Sonography is operator dependent and limited by abdominal wall thickness. It is not a good modality for evaluation of diaphragmatic, pancreatic, and bowel injuries and bony pelvis. Finally, sonography in some studies has failed to demonstrate or has been false-negative in roughly 25–33% of solid organ injuries [7].

Focused assessment with sonography for trauma (FAST) is a rapid examination of abdominal and lower thoracic region performed as a part of preliminary evaluation of patients with suspected abdominal trauma with blunt abdominal or thoracic injuries. This is mainly to search for intraperitoneal fluid. It is basically a six-point study best performed with 3.5 MHz small footprint sector transducer. A quick examination with recording of longitudinal and transverse images in the following areas should be done in the right subdiaphragmatic space, the left subdiaphragmatic space, the hepatorenal recess, the perisplenic space, the pelvic peritoneal recess, and the pericardium. FAST is primarily aimed at detection of hemoperitoneum, while parenchymal solid organ injuries may be detected, but negative FAST basically implies the absence of hemoperitoneum and not the absence of intra-abdominal injury [8]. Because of its relatively low sensitivity, FAST is not equivalent to CT. Hemodynamically stable patients with positive FAST should have further evaluation of injuries with computed tomography [8].

7.6   Contrast-Enhanced Ultrasound

In the last decade, a new addition to ultrasonographic technique has been developed using contrast agents (USCAs). Contrast-enhanced ultrasound (CEUS) has many advantages over routine ultrasonography for the detection of abdominal injuries. It remains to be seen whether it has significant utility in clinical scenarios in India beyond its research utility.

7.6.1   Agents

The ultrasound contrast agents (USCAs) used are sulfur hexafluoride or perfluorocarbon encapsulated in a phospholipid outer shell and stabilized as gas microbubbles of 1–7 μm. These bubbles remain in circulation and on transmission of ultrasonic wave generate a harmonic nonlinear reaction that can be distinguished from the tissue signal. The contrast microbubbles remain mainly in vessels—in large and small vessels. This feature of ultrasound contrast agent is utilized by specially developed software in ultrasound machines that enable delineation of signal between the main tissue and gas-filled microbubbles of contrast agents. As soon as the bolus of contrast agent is injected in a peripheral vein, the arterial phase starts the moment microbubbles enter the arterial end, and they remain in circulation until their dissolution. This allows prompt and continuous depiction of the lesion for a longer time irrespective of phase. This is unlike CT and MR where sequences have to be planned and timed at the height of enhancement for each phase which can lead to missed focal injuries due to inaccurate timing. Moreover, the echogenicity of the surrounding parenchyma is not affected in contrast ultrasound imaging.

In trauma patients, contrast ultrasound should be performed only after conventional ultrasound imaging as the utility of conventional ultrasound in complete evaluation cannot be overemphasized. It can be performed by using contrast pulse sequence imaging or by using pulse inversion harmonic imaging [7–9]. The contrast agent is given as a fast bolus injection through the antecubital vein or other accessible peripheral veins. The injuries involving vessels tend to appear within 1 min of contrast administration, and parenchymal solid organ injuries are demonstrated for a longer time during all the phases till the contrast persists in circulation.

7.7 Adverse Reactions and Contraindications

USCAs are usually well-tolerated drugs and very rarely any severe reactions are seen. Contraindications include heart failure, septal defects with right left shunting, angina pectoris, pregnancy, and breastfeeding [10, 11].

USCAs are not nephrotoxic and can be used safely in patients with acute or chronic renal insufficiency and do not interact with the adrenals, pancreas, or thyroid gland hormones.

Contrast-enhanced US is clearly a very useful adjunct to conventional ultrasound imaging especially in diagnosing the number and the size of intraperitoneal solid organ injuries or retroperitoneal injuries. It can disclose probable capsular involvement and can reveal the presence of related vascular injuries suggested by contrast extravasation, parenchymal infarction, and vascular avulsion. The solid organ injuries are shown as nonenhancing defects, while lacerations and contusion areas and the lesions involving parenchyma appear inhomogeneous anechoic or hypoechoic areas without mass effect. Active bleeding and pseudoaneurysms are diagnosed when there is extravasation of microbubbles into the parenchyma or as collections around viscera [11].

However at times significant injuries may be missed by the sonologist. Small parenchymal injuries may be missed, especially in multi-trauma setting, and obesity at times may be an issue or when the hematoma is small. Overall view and complete assessment of intra-abdominal organs are better with conventional ultrasound imaging than contrast ultrasound. Injuries to the collecting system of the kidney are more likely to be missed on CEUS due to lack of microbubble visualization in urinary excretion. Post-traumatic ileus with large amount of bowel gas may also prove a hindrance in visualization [12, 13].

7.8 CT Scan

CT scan is the modality of choice in the hemodynamically stable patient [14, 15]. CT is able to detect abdominal injuries with accuracy, is noninvasive, and is usually the preferred imaging modality consistent with conservative management in pediatric abdominal trauma, but it is comparatively expensive and endangers the child to ionizing radiation exposure [16].

7.8.1 Indications

Abdominal CT scan is usually performed if:

1. The patient is stable hemodynamically.
2. No definite indications or injury requiring urgent emergency procedures.
3. No obvious signs of peritonitis or free air on plain radiograph of the abdomen [17, 18].

7.8.2   Procedure and Protocol

Abdominal CT is performed right from the diaphragm to the pubic symphysis. Scans are usually taken at 1 cm intervals but are adjusted according to the age and size of the child [17, 18]. A nonionic dimer contrast material is used for intravenous injection at a dose of 2 mL/kg. In performing CT scan with blunt trauma, the use of both intravenous and oral contrast media is necessary. Water-soluble contrast material is administered in dilution through the oral or nasogastric tube about 30–40 min before CT scanning and an additional amount just before the scanning. In addition to soft tissue window settings, lung window and bone window settings are essential in looking out for extraluminal air or bone fractures.

7.8.3   Consideration of Radiation Exposure

Although the issue of radiation exposure comes only as an afterthought in the minds of radiologists and trauma surgeons in scanning of acute trauma victims, it is an important issue to consider in the evaluation of children. This is because the tissues of children have more of rapidly dividing cells and also because the long latent period for radiation-induced malignancies makes them more likely to manifest during the future life span of a child than in an adult or old patient. The parameters—peak kilovoltage (KVp), tube current (mAs), pitch, and section thickness—should be planned as regards the child's body size and weight, keeping in view the principles of ALARA (as low as reasonably achievable) and also ensuring at the same time that no diagnostic information is lost in doing so.

7.8.4   Interpretation of Scans

The most commonly injured solid intra-abdominal organ is the liver followed by the spleen [19, 20].

7.8.4.1 Hepatic Injury

Most of the hepatic injuries involve the posterior segment of the right lobe [20]. The features seen on CT are periportal low-attenuation tracking, subcapsular and parenchymal hematomas, lacerations, contusions, and active bleeding. Subcapsular hematoma appear as concavo-convex hypoattenuating collections between the capsule of the liver and liver parenchyma on contrast-enhanced CT (CECT). Parenchymal hematomas appear as focal areas of low attenuation in the liver parenchyma on contrast-enhanced CT. Actually attenuation value depends on the time since the bleed, acute hematomas being hyperattenuated (40–60 HU) compared to normal liver tissue on unenhanced CT [17]. Lacerations involving the liver appear as irregular branching or linear low-attenuation areas on CECT (Fig. 7.1). Active hemorrhage is seen as a collection of hyperattenuated (91–274 Hounsfield units) extravasated contrast material on early phase-enhanced CT [15]. On CT, bile duct injuries have a nonspecific appearance and may appear as simple lacerations of the

Fig. 7.1 CECT abdomen image showing large hepatic laceration with hematoma—Grade 3 liver injury

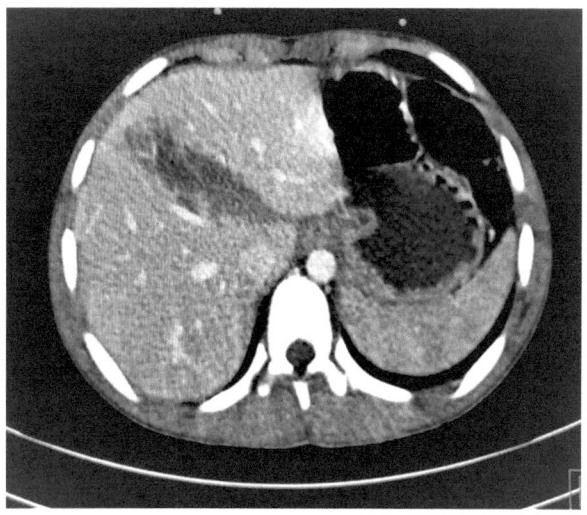

liver or localized collections around bile ducts. For exact diagnosis, hepatobiliary scintigraphy is indicated to show active extravasation of bile at the site of duct injury [21–23]. The grading of liver injury by the American Association of Surgeons for Trauma (AAST) scale grades injuries into six grades [21]:

Grade 1: haematoma: subcapsular (<10% surface area), laceration: capsular tear (<1 cm parenchymal depth).

Grade 2: haematoma: subcapsular (10-50% surface area), haematoma: intraparenchymal (<10 cm diameter), laceration: capsular tear 1-3 cm, parenchymal depth <10 cm length.

Grade 3: haematoma: subcapsular (>50% surface area) or parenchymal haematoma, haematoma: intraparenchymal >10 cm or expanding, laceration: capsular tear >3 cm parenchymal depth.

Grade 4: laceration: parenchymal disruption involving 25–75% hepatic lobe or involves 1–3 Couinaud segments (Fig. 7.2).

Grade 5: laceration: parenchymal disruption involving >75% of hepatic lobe or involves >3 Couinaud segments (within one lobe), vascular: juxtahepatic venous injuries (retrohepatic vena cava / central major hepatic veins).

Grade 6: vascular hepatic avulsion *Advance one grade for multiple injuries upto grade III.

The AAST grading of liver injury as well as the hemodynamic status should be considered in the management of liver injuries of a child [22]. Patients with higher grade of liver injury and continuous bleeding and shock despite aggressive blood and fluid transfusion may need exploratory laparotomy. A hemodynamically stable child having lower grade of injury must be managed conservatively with close surgical supervision.

Fig. 7.2 CECT image showing right lobar destruction of the liver with a large hematoma— Grade 4 liver injury

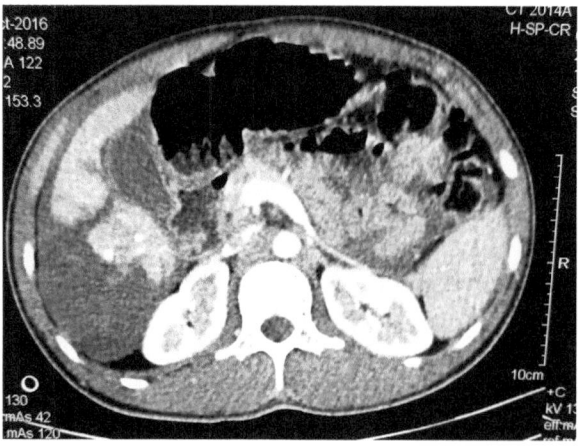

7.8.4.2 Splenic Injury

The spleen is the second most common injured solid organ in the abdomen in children with blunt injuries [19]. A child with left upper quadrant pain or tenderness, left lower chest or upper abdominal contusion, or fracture of left lower ribs should be suspected to have splenic injury. These children are mainly managed conservatively because of the risk of infection and sepsis after splenectomy [1]. The indication for splenectomy in children is massive disruption of the spleen with hemodynamic instability and shock [22]. The AAST grading of spleen injury is as follows [21]:

Grade 1: hematoma (subcapsular) <10% of surface area or tear in capsule involving <1 cm depth

Grade 2: hematoma (subcapsular) between 10 and 50% of surface area, hematoma in parenchyma, hematoma of size <5 cm in diameter, or parenchymal laceration of 1–3 cm in depth

Grade 3: hematoma (subcapsular) of >50% of surface area or expanding and ruptured subcapsular or parenchymal hematoma, intraparenchymal hematoma of more than 5 cm, or laceration of more than 3 cm in depth

Grade 4: laceration involving segmental or hilar vessels with devascularization of more than 1/4 of the spleen

Grade 5: shattered spleen or hilar vascular injury *Advance one grade for multiple injuries upto grade III

A subcapsular hematoma has a concavo-convex shape flattening the adjacent spleen surface. Splenic laceration is seen as an irregular branching or linear hypoattenuating area in the spleen associated with fluid in the abdomen (Fig. 7.3). The fluid may have a higher CT value as it represents hemoperitoneum.

Fig. 7.3 Grade 3 splenic injury with laceration and hematoma on CT

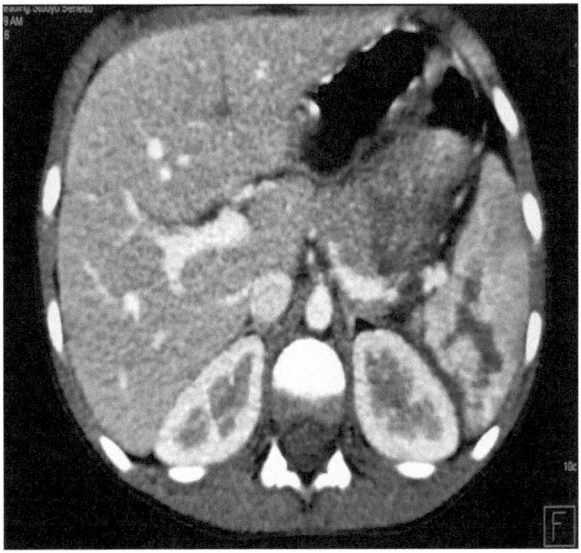

7.8.4.3 Renal Trauma

Children with renal trauma present with flank tenderness and/or hematuria. After screening with USG, CT should be used for complete evaluation. Subcapsular hematomas, hematomas, and lacerations have the same appearance as described in spleen and liver injury. The presence of contrast enhancement within a laceration or around the renal fossa through the pyelographic phase of the CT examination indicates the injury to collecting system [19]. It is important to look for pelvicalyceal system injury and urinary leakage by taking delayed scan in excretory phase. Excretory phase-enhanced CT of the renal system is performed 3 min after injection of contrast agent. It is necessary for complete assessment of a suspected injury to renal parenchyma as well as the collecting system injury [24].

The AAST grading of renal injury is [21]:

- Grade I: contusion or non-enlarging subcapsular perirenal haematoma or normal urologic studies in presence of microscopic or gross hematuria.
- Grade II: superficial laceration <1 cm depth and does not reach the pelvicalyceal system; non-expanding perirenal hematoma confined to retroperitoneum.
- Grade III: laceration >1 cm, without extension into the renal pelvis or collecting system.
- Grade IV: laceration extends to renal pelvis or urinary extravasation or vascular injury to main renal artery or vein with contained haemorrhage or segmental infarctions without associated lacerations.
- Grade V: shattered kidney or renal hilum avulsion or ureteropelvic avulsion or complete laceration or thrombus of the main renal artery or vein (Fig. 7.4).
 *Advance one grade for bilateral injuries up to grade III

Fig. 7.4 CECT image
showing shattered right
kidney with large
perinephric hematoma

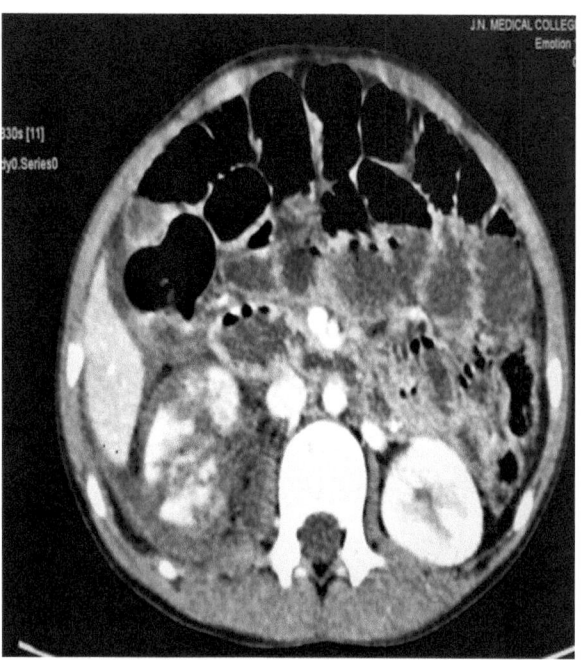

7.8.4.4 Pancreatic and Other Solid Organ Injury

Pancreatic injury is uncommon in blunt trauma abdomen compared to other commonly injured organs discussed above. Because it is less suspected, its diagnosis is easily missed and may lead to complications and increased morbidity. Major frequency of injuries occurs in the pancreatic body, and most of these injuries are associated with injury to other solid and hollow viscera like the liver, spleen, stomach, and duodenum. Isolated pancreatic injury is rare [25]. CT features suggesting pancreatic injury are thickened pancreas, peripancreatic fat stranding, peripancreatic fluid, and fluid between the splenic vein and pancreatic parenchyma [25]. Complete transection of the pancreas may also occur in rare circumstances (Fig. 7.5). CT findings may be supported by lab evidence of pancreatic enzyme elevation. The prognosis for pancreatic trauma is good if recognized early because majority of injuries can be managed conservatively; however delayed complications are likely. Adrenal glands may also be injured in very rare circumstances, either isolated or in association with other injuries.

7.8.4.5 Injury to Bowel and Mesentery

Although intestinal injury following blunt abdominal trauma is uncommon, when present, it can be quite significant if it remains undiagnosed or misdiagnosed for even few hours. Even though the accuracy of CT is controversial, CT (particularly helical CT) is effective in detecting mesenteric and bowel injury in blunt abdominal

Fig. 7.5 Pancreatic laceration at the neck of the pancreas with peripancreatic and perihepatic collection

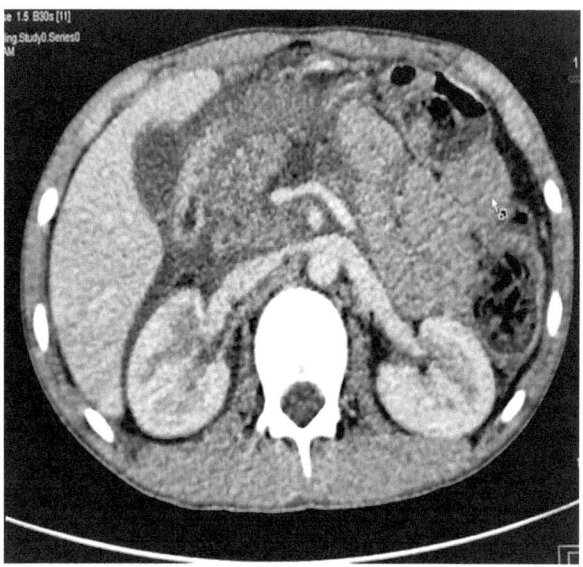

trauma and is very useful in deciding whether surgical repair or conservative management is needed [25]. While performing CT scan in a child with blunt trauma and suspected bowel or mesenteric injury, the use of both intravenous and oral contrast media is necessary. Water-soluble contrast material with adequate dilution is administered periorally or through the nasogastric tube about 30–40 min before CT scanning and an additional small amount just before the scanning. Scans are usually taken at 1 cm slice gap from the dome of diaphragm to the level of pubic symphysis throughout the abdomen. In addition to soft tissue window settings, lung window and bone window settings are essential in looking out for extraluminal air or bone fractures. The most specific signs of a bowel injury are frank extravasation of oral contrast media and pneumoperitoneum or retroperitoneal air. However, these signs especially the extravasation of oral contrast media are seen only in few cases of bowel injury. Intraperitoneal gas may also be seen as a result of causes other than bowel perforation as pneumomediastinum or diagnostic peritoneal lavage. Other less specific signs of bowel injury include:

(a) Peritoneal fluid especially interloop or triangular fluid collections provided solid organ injury or rupture of urinary bladder is excluded
(b) Sentinel clot sign which indicates high-attenuation heterogeneous clot near the site of injury [26]
(c) Focal bowel wall thickening or bowel wall discontinuity
(d) Intense contrast enhancement of bowel wall
(e) Adjacent mesenteric hematoma or infiltration (streaky density)

In mesenteric injury, extravasation of intravenous contrast media indicates vascular compromise of bowel or continued hemorrhage mandating surgical exploration

[16, 26]. CT may miss some cases of bowel injury; such cases require careful clinical observation, follow-up CT scan, DPL, or even surgical exploration [14].

7.8.5 Avoiding Pitfalls in Diagnosis

Pitfalls may result in false-positive and false-negative diagnoses of injury. It is important to view the scans in lung window and bone window settings in addition to soft tissue window settings to avoid missing extraluminal air-pneumoperitoneum in bowel perforation or bone fractures. It is also important to use both intravenous and oral contrast media in suspected bowel injury to look for extravasation of oral contrast media—one of the definite signs of bowel perforation. Congenital variants like splenic clefts may mimic a laceration, but they have more smooth margins, while a laceration has irregular margins. Non-contrast images are useful when looking for active bleed which appear as increased attenuation areas in non-enhanced organ; this finding may be missed if only contrast-enhanced scanning is performed. Heterogeneous enhancement of the liver, spleen, and kidneys immediately after contrast administration also needs to be interpreted with caution.

7.8.6 Role of CT Scan in Follow-Up

The role of repeat CT scans has increased considerably with the conservative management of injuries.

The size of contusions and hematomas, laceration, and amount of hemoperitoneum need to be followed up closely in every patient. Scanning may also need to be repeated to check postoperative repair. However all this makes radiation protection measures more imperative.

7.9 Magnetic Resonance Imaging (MRI)

Abdominal MRI is an imaging modality with diverse armamentarium and excellent soft tissue contrast enhancement including the T1, T2, HASTE, trueFISP, and dynamic contrast-enhanced imaging. But because of its cost constraints and relative inaccessibility in remote areas, it is not used in the assessment of acutely injured patient. However after the initial imaging or in postoperative period or follow-up, the role of MRI comes up when better cross-sectional imaging is required [27].

Angiography sequences are used to evaluate for arterial-venous fistulas or malformations in the follow-up that may develop following trauma. MRCP provides superior noninvasive evaluation of the biliary system following trauma. In addition, certain hepatocyte-specific MRI contrast agents have been developed as gadolinium-BOPTA (MultiHance) and gadolinium-EOB-DTPA (Primovist), which provide excellent details of the biliary system anatomy (strictures or bile leaks). MRI can also help in differentiating seroma and biloma collections in the abdomen. MRI has also been found to be very useful in the evaluation of pancreatic injuries especially when conservative management is planned. MRCP allows better visualization and delineation of anatomy of bile ducts. In children where multiple follow-ups are required, MR plays an important role by minimizing cumulative radiation dose.

References

1. Eklof O. Abdominal plain film diagnosis in infants and children. Progr Pediatr Radiol. 1969;2:3.
2. Frimann-Dahl J. Roentgen examinations in acute abdominal diseases. 3rd ed. Springfield: Charles Thomas; 1974.
3. Jorulf H. Roentgen diagnosis of intraperitoneal fluid. Acta Radiol. 1975;343(Suppl. 343):85.
4. Fischer KC, Eraklis A, Treves S. Scintigraphy in the follow-up of pediatric splenic trauma treated without surgery. J Nucl Med. 1978;19:3–9.
5. Griffin LH Jr, Garrison AF, Ihnen M. Influence of radioisotope imaging on current treatment of blunt splenic trauma. Am Surg. 1978;44:318.
6. Lang EK. Arteriography in the assessment of renal trauma. J Trauma. 1975;15:554–66.
7. Richards JR, Knopf NA, Wang L, McGahan JP. Blunt abdominal trauma in children: Evaluation with emergency US. Emerg Radiol. 2002;222(3):749–54.
8. Chiu WC, Cushing BM, Rodriguez A, et al. Abdominal injuries without hemoperitoneum: A potential limitation of focused abdominal sonography for trauma (FAST). J Trauma. 1997;42(4):617–23.
9. Cokkinos D, Antypa K, Stefanidis K, et al. Contrast-enhanced ultrasound for imaging blunt abdominal trauma – indication, description of the technique and imaging review. Ultraschall in Med. 2012;33:60–7.
10. Valentino M, Serra C, Zironi G, et al. Blunt abdominal trauma: Emergency contrast-enhanced sonography for detection of solid organ injuries. AJR. 2006;186:1361–7.
11. Valentino M, Serra C, Pavlica P, et al. Contrast-enhanced ultrasound for blunt abdominal trauma. Semin Ultrasound CT MR. 2007;28(2):130–40.
12. Esposito F, Di Serafino M, Sgambati P, Mercogliano F, Tarantino L, Vallone G, Oresta P. Ultrasound contrast media in paediatric patients: Is it an off-label use? Regulatory requirements and radiologist's liability. Radiol Med. 2012;117(1):148–59.
13. Stylianos S. Outcomes from pediatric solid organ injury: Role of standardized care guidelines. Curr Opin Pediatr. 2005;17:402–6.
14. Strouse PJ, Close BJ, Marshall KW, Cywes R. CT of bowel and mesenteric trauma in children. Radiographics. 1999;19(5):1237–50.
15. Wegner S, Colletti JE, Van Wie D. Pediatric blunt abdominal trauma. Pediatr Clin North Am. 2006;53:243–56.
16. Holmes JF, Sokolove PE, Brant WE, et al. Identification of children with intra-abdominal injuries after blunt trauma. Ann Emerg Med. 2002;39:500–9.
17. Ruess L, Sivit CJ, Eichelberger MR, et al. Blunt hepatic and splenic trauma in children: Correlation of a CT injury severity scale with clinical outcome. Pediatr Radiol. 1995;25:321–5.
18. Potoka DA, Saladino RA. Blunt abdominal trauma in the pediatric patient. Clin Ped Emerg Med. 2005;6:23–31.
19. West OC, Jarolimek AM. Abdomen- traumatic emergencies. In: Harris JH, Harris WH, editors. The radiology of emergency medicine. 4th ed. Philadelphia: Lippincott Williams & Wilkins; 2000. p. 689–723.
20. Eppich WJ, Zonfrillo MR. Emergency department evaluation and management of blunt abdominal trauma in children. Curr Opin Pediatr. 2007;19:265–9.
21. Moore EE, Cogbill TH, Malangoni MA, et al. Organ injury scaling. Surg Clin North Am. 1995;75(2):293–303.

22. Sivit CJ, Frazier AA, Eichelberger MR. Computed tomography of pediatric blunt abdominal trauma. Emerg Radiol. 1997;4:150–66.
23. Yoon W, Jeong YY, Kim JK, et al. CT in blunt liver trauma. Radiographics. 2005;25:87–104.
24. Ramchandani P, Buckler PM. Imaging of genitourinary trauma. AJR Am J Roentgenol. 2009;192(6):1514–23.
25. Gupta A, Stuhlfaut JW, Fleming KW, Lucey BC, Soto JA. Blunt trauma of the pancreas and biliary tract: A multimodality imaging approach to diagnosis. Radiographics. 2004;24:1381–95.
26. Sherek J, Shatney C, Sensaki K, et al. The accuracy of computed tomography in the diagnosis of blunt small bowel perforation. Am J of Surg. 1994;168:670–5.
27. Tkacz JN, Anderson SA, Soto J. MR imaging in gastrointestinal emergencies. Radiographics. 2009;29(6):1767–80.

Interventional Imaging in Pediatric Abdominal Trauma

8

Shagufta Wahab

The most common form of treatment of abdominal injuries in children is conservative, and it depends on the child's response to initial resuscitation. However, a small percentage of children with blunt abdominal trauma may be nonresponsive to blood and fluid resuscitation due to significant injury with continuous internal bleeding. Such a patient requires emergent surgical or interventional radiology intervention to prevent hemorrhagic shock. Surgical exploration of unknown bleeding point could become even lengthier if the injury requires repair. This is not desirable in the aforementioned clinical scenario. Here comes the role of angiography and selective transarterial embolization/stenting in "damage control" and salvaging the patient. Thus in the acute bleeding, interventional radiology may help to control the hemorrhage or reestablish blood flow by using stents. In elective setting, it can help percutaneous stenting and drainage of urinary and biliary systems. Interventional radiology can also come as a rescue in the management of delayed complications of trauma, e.g., fistulas or pseudoaneurysms [1, 2].

8.1 Indications

1. In hemodynamically unstable patients, it is used as a minimally invasive technique to stop bleeding by transarterial embolization or stent grafting.
2. Management of solid organ injuries.
3. Placing percutaneous drains or stents in injury to hepatobiliary apparatus or renal collecting system.

S. Wahab
Department of Radiodiagnosis, Jawaharlal Nehru Medical College, AMU, Aligarh, Uttar Pradesh, India

© Springer Nature Singapore Pte Ltd. 2018
R. Ahmad Khan, S. Wahab (eds.), *Blunt Abdominal Trauma in Children*,
https://doi.org/10.1007/978-981-13-0692-1_8

8.2   Interventional Radiology (IR) Technique

The basic aim of an IR procedure should be to definitively control hemorrhage with limited intervention so that the patient is stabilized. The final reconstructive procedure or redo intervention measures should be performed after the patient is stabilized. While controlling the bleeding by embolization, it should be kept in mind that embolization is performed in the distal most bleeding vessel source as possible to decrease the amount of parenchymal damage and accumulation of anaerobic metabolites including lactic acid [1, 2].

In children the dose of contrast medium is 3–5 ml/kg. Since this is generally followed by saline flush, it should be emphasized that the total amount of saline volume given should be titrated minutely in babies and toddlers to circumvent accidental overload.

Acquiring vascular access in children in shock especially with small vessels may be a difficult task. The vascular access should be guided by ultrasound or fluoroscopy wherever available. Most commonly vascular access in children is achieved through the femoral vein or artery. The size of the sheath depends on patients' age and size as well as the vessel in which intervention is planned. Generally in infants less than 12 kg, a 3F sheath is preferred and while in majority 4F sheath. The most common embolizing agents used are metal coils and biodegradable gelatin sponge particles [3, 4].

8.2.1   Liver

Mostly liver injuries with extensive hemorrhage are managed with packing.

High-grade hepatic injuries may cause widespread damage to vascular and biliary structures that may manifest as delayed complications of treatment like recurrent hemorrhage, bile leaks, pseudoaneurysms, etc. Frequently hepatic necrosis is seen after embolization, leading to abscess formation within the liver parenchyma that may require percutaneous drainage. This necessitates that embolization should be done as selective as possible. Fistulas and pseudoaneurysms should be coiled as distally as is sufficient to stop the bleed.

Bile duct leaks and bilomas are frequently managed by percutaneous drainage or stent placement. This can be achieved percutaneously or by endoscopic retrograde cholangiopancreatography (ERCP). A combined approach, using percutaneous procedure and guided by flouroscopy or ultrasonography from above and simultaneous ERCP from below is used to repair the damaged ducts [5].

8.2.2   Spleen

The spleen is frequently injured in abdominal trauma and significant hemorrhage may occur from a disrupted spleen. Splenectomy was the typical treatment for a badly injured spleen. However, following splenectomy, children have weakened immunity against many encapsulated bacteria particularly pneumococcus and are predisposed to frequent attacks of pneumonia. Hence conservative management is now the main mode of management. In extensive disruption of the spleen, embolization of the proximal splenic artery can be done to decrease the blood flow to the spleen and hence to reduce intrasplenic pressure within the capsule so that healing occurs without significant ischemia or infarction as the short gastric and other vessels maintain the necessary collateral supply of blood [6, 7].

Several studies have reported that in hemodynamically stable patients, embolization reduces mortality without splenectomy.

8.2.3   Pancreas

Pancreatic trauma may lead to pseudocyst formation when percutaneous drainage under CT guidance is frequently performed. Transgastric approach rather than percutaneous is also recommended by others [8, 9].

8.2.4   Genitourinary System

Renal vessel injuries frequently occur in association with other solid organ injuries and require embolization. Again this should be performed as selective as possible decreasing renal parenchymal damage. This may obviate the need of nephrectomy altogether or at least it may be delayed after initial hemostasis is achieved. Delayed complications like fistulas or pseudoaneurysms can be embolized with coils or biodegradable gelatin sponge pledgets.

Disruption of renal collecting system may lead to urinoma formation which may become secondarily infected. Percutaneous drainage of these collections and placement of percutaneous nephrostomy tube significantly improve the condition of these severely sick children and can be easily performed under ultrasound guidance as an outpatient procedure. Once the condition improves, collecting system repair can be done by placement of ureteral stents. Urethral obstruction following urethral injury or bladder outlet obstruction or leak may require placement of a suprapubic cystostomy catheter under fluoroscopy. Foley catheter can also be placed under ultrasonography where over-the-wire placement of catheter is done to drain the bladder [10, 11].

8.2.5   Major Vessel Injuries

Injury to aorta following blunt abdominal trauma in children is uncommon; however this may occur in high-velocity road traffic accidents. Multidetector CT is the principal imaging modality for appropriate diagnosis. Management of aortic injuries may require placement of a stent across the site of vessel wall damage or transection to avert the emergency need of aortic repair [2–4].

8.2.6 Pelvis

Blunt or penetrating trauma affecting pelvis may lead to uncontrolled bleeding which may not be easily amenable to surgical exploration. The bleeding may be from one of the pelvic vessels or bone. Surgery may exacerbate the bleeding by taking off the tamponade effect of fascial planes. Transcatheter endovascular embolization is now a well-established technique for uncontrolled pelvic arterial bleeding. Early complication of embolization may cause skin necrosis, ulceration, or nerve injury, while delayed complications may produce claudication and local pain. Straddle injury in children may lead to injury to pudendal artery and resultant priapism. In these cases, embolization of pudendal artery improves priapism [2].

8.2.7 Inferior Vena Cava (IVC) Filter

Trauma patients are frequently bed ridden for long periods which makes them susceptible to deep venous thrombosis (DVT). In these patients IVC filters are indicated. Other patients who need IVC filter are those in whom anticoagulation drugs cannot be started due to initial injury or ongoing surgical procedures. IVC filters may be placed via a jugular or femoral approach. Filters are ideally placed just below the renal veins. Filter removal is either via a jugular approach or femoral approach depending on the filter type [2, 4].

Thus, in children of blunt abdominal trauma with hemodynamic instability and shock interventional radiology (IR), techniques have the potential to replace surgery and prove to be a life savior. It can also limit collateral parenchymal damage. It is also an important tool in the management of patients with delayed complications associated with trauma or its conservative/surgical treatment. However there are many factors that preclude the extensive use of this technique in children, including (1) widely variable pediatric age range, (2) differing etiologies of pediatric trauma, (3) equipment that is too large to accommodate small pediatric blood vessels, and (4) experience or comfort level in treating children. Despite these reasons, interventional radiologists' role in pediatric trauma is increasing. This is attributed to increasing experience and development of newer age equipment, microcatheters, and coils.

References

1. Kiankhooy A, Sartorelli KH, Vane DW, Bhave AD. Angiographic embolization is safe and effective therapy for blunt abdominal solid organ injury in children. J Trauma. 2010;68:526–31.
2. Vo NJ, Althoen M, Hippe DS, Prabhu SJ, Valji K, Padia SA. Pediatric abdominal and pelvic trauma: safety and efficacy of arterial embolization. J Vasc Interv Radiol. 2014;25:215–20.
3. Wahlgren CM, Kragsterman B. Management and outcomes of pediatric vascular injuries. J Trauma Acute Care Surg. 2015;79:563–7.
4. Rowland SP, Dharmarajah B, Moore HM, et al. Venous injuries in pediatric trauma: systematic review of injuries and management. J Trauma Acute Care Surg. 2014;77:356–63.

5. Lee YH, Wu CH, Wang LJ, Wong YC, Chen HW, Wang CJ, et al. Predictive factors for early failure of transarterial embolization in blunt hepatic injury patients. Clin Radiol. 2014;69:e505–11.
6. Gross JL, Woll NL, Hanson CA, et al. Embolization for pediatric blunt splenic injury in an alternative to splenectomy when observation fails. J Trauma Acute Care Surg. 2013;75:421–5.
7. Gaarder C, Dormagen JB, Eken T, Skaga NO, Klow NE, Pillgram-Larsen J, et al. Nonoperative management of splenic injuries: improved results with angioembolization. J Trauma. 2006;61:192–8.
8. Boudghene F, L'Hennine C, Bigot J. Arterial complications of pancreatitis: diagnostic and therapeutic aspects in 104 cases. J Vasc Interv Radiol. 1993;4:551–8.
9. Mauro MA, Jaques P. Transcatheter management of pseudoaneurysms complicating pancreatitis. J Vasc Interv Radiol. 1991;2:527–32.
10. Wessel LM, Scholz S, Jester I, Arnold R, Lorenz C, Hosie S, et al. Management of kidney injuries in children with blunt abdominal trauma. J Pediatr Surg. 2000;35(9):1326–30.
11. Margenthaler JA, Weber TR, Keller MS. Blunt renal trauma in children: experience with conservative management at a pediatric trauma center. J Trauma. 2002;52:928–32.

Anesthetic and Critical Care Considerations in Children with Abdominal Trauma

Lalit Gupta and Bhavna Gupta

9.1 Introduction

Unrecognized abdominal trauma is a common unrecognized life-threatening emergency on pediatric age group. As compared to adults, children have large solid organs; they have low subcutaneous fat and have no significantly low abdominal muscle mass to protect. Solid organ injuries are common in children due to blunt and penetrating trauma. Blunt trauma causes injury to solid organs such as the liver and spleen. The potentially life-threatening injuries are real challenge to the attending anesthesiologist as the children are not only anatomically and physiologically different from adult but also psychologically more difficult to deal with [1, 2].

Like any traumatic injury, priority in children presented in emergency with trauma includes not only recognition of compromised airway and prompt relief but also immediate measures for unforeseen injuries to cervical spine. Other domains that needs immediate attention are chest injuries (often life-threatening) and shock. Sometimes major intra-abdominal bleeding is masked despite significant blood loss because of physiological tendency of children to maintain normal blood pressure till late. The examining intensivist must remember that the peritoneal cavity is a large potential reservoir for blood loss, and hence blunt trauma to the abdomen should be attended with utmost care.

L. Gupta (✉) · B. Gupta
Department of Anesthesia and Critical Care, Maulana Azad Medical College,
New Delhi, India

© Springer Nature Singapore Pte Ltd. 2018
R. Ahmad Khan, S. Wahab (eds.), *Blunt Abdominal Trauma in Children*,
https://doi.org/10.1007/978-981-13-0692-1_9

9.2   Pediatric Airway and Breathing

9.2.1   Airway

Airway in children is far anatomically different from an adult's airway. Large tongue may lead to an unnoticed airway obstruction and difficult laryngoscopy. There is anterior and cephalad placement of the larynx, and the epiglottis is shorter and omega shaped, leading to difficult intubation. Angulation of vocal cords in relation to laryngeal inlet often leads to lodging of endotracheal tube in anterior commissure. Relatively large head and short neck in children again contribute to challenging laryngoscopic position, especially if rigid cervical collar is in place. Large occiput in children causes auto-flexion of cervical spine leading to airway obstruction on lying flat. Proportionally large tongue in relation to narrow oropharynx may obstruct the airway under anesthesia. Therefore, proper jaw positioning enables bag and mask ventilation until trachea is intubated. There is risk of gaseous distension of the abdomen and aspiration of gastric contents if ventilation is done through an obstructed airway. Cervical spine injury may be common in children due to flexible interspinous ligaments, anterior wedging of vertebral bodies, and tendency to slide forward with flexion owing to flat facet joint. The actual incidence of cervical injuries is comparatively less in children than in adults. But until the spinal injury is thoroughly excluded by examination, the neck should be immobilized with appropriate support. Rigid cervical collar is always preferred for it with patient immobilized on a spine board. Soft collars are usually ineffective for immobilizing the neck [2].

9.2.2   Breathing

After establishing an airway, adequacy of respiration should be ensured by observation of symmetric chest movement, a five-point auscultation of chest, and a chest X-ray. Establishment of a patent airway always remains as first priority.

Noisy or labored respiration or paradoxical respiration is evidence of airway obstruction. All efforts should be made to remove vomitus, blood, or foreign matter from the mouth either manually or by means of sucker. Chin lift and jaw thrust are simple yet effective measure which prevents tongue from falling backward, thus preventing obstruction in unconscious patients [2, 3].

Appropriate-sized oropharyngeal and nasopharyngeal airways are adjuncts to relieve airway obstruction. Tension hemopneumothorax can be diagnosed clinically and treated by needle aspiration. This maneuver will not only alleviate the tension but also gains time till a chest tube can be inserted.

9.3   Circulation and Fluid Resuscitation in Children [4, 5]

Circulation in a child is assessed by following parameters:

- Sudden and marked tachycardia
- Compromised peripheral perfusion

- Weakly palpable peripheral pulses
- Hypotension (present when >25% of circulating blood volume is lost)
- Presence of sign and symptoms of shock

If possible central line cannulation should be rapidly done in a child who is severely hypovolemic. Intraosseous line should be chosen if one is unable to place a peripheral venous catheter. Volume resuscitation is judged by clinical condition of the child, estimated blood, or plasma volume lost during trauma.

1. *Shock* is a metabolic derangement in body where oxygen supply is unable to meet oxygen demand due to metabolic derangements at various levels. In a child with several injuries entailing surgical intervention, it is imperative to assess fluid status quickly before any intervention is done. Anesthesiologist and intensivist should maintain the resuscitation if there is continuing blood loss or third space losses. The goal of resuscitation is to sustain normovolemia and maintenance of normal osmolar and oncotic pressures.
2. Vital parameters are age-dependent. A minimum of 15% of circulating blood volume loss must be there for signs of shock to manifest clinically in children. Hypotension is seen when there is acute loss of 25% of circulating blood volume. Twenty milliliter per kilogram isotonic saline is administered when there are signs of shock, and the same can be repeated as desired. This initial resuscitation volume must be equivalent to minimum of 25% of the circulating volume, while second bolus resuscitation must comprise of volume equivalent to 50% of the circulating volume. Isotonic crystalloids such as ringer lactate or normal saline are the most preferred solutions in initial stages of resuscitation. Symptoms and signs of shock can be non-specific; some children may just present with a non-specific sign of tachycardia which is often confused with signs of pain or discomfort. Unlike adults, systolic pressure can be increased in pediatric age group.
3. Some authors advocate the use of hypertonic saline solutions as they are supposed to increase serum osmolality and retain fluid in intravascular compartment for longer periods with lesser volume of the solution administered as compared to isotonic solutions. However, this has not been corroborated with large cohort study. Glucose-containing fluids must be given with great caution if there is an associated head trauma, since elevated blood glucose levels are associated with poor neurologic outcomes in pediatric age group.
4. Colloid solutions which include 5% albumin and hydroxyethyl starch (HES) may be used for resuscitation, but there are concerns of exacerbation of coagulopathy because of the use of HES. They are known to affect platelet function, decrease fibrinogen activity, and interfere with factor VIII activity also.
5. Nevertheless, they are the preferred agents in victims of head trauma, owing to their ability to increase colloid osmotic pressure and relatively smaller volume required to produce desired beneficial effects than crystalloids. They may also reduce the incidence of cerebral edema in children with head trauma.

9.4   Transfusion and Its Indications

9.4.1   Blood Product Transfusion

Blood transfusion is given to maintain oxygen delivery and to establish hemostasis in pediatric cases with trauma. Packed red cells are given to meet the oxygen-carrying capacity with that of tissue demands and metabolic rate. Crystalloids and colloids are given to replace up to 40% of losses of blood volumes without much compromising upon oxygen. For loses >40%, blood transfusion should be the first choice without further delay. The decision is also governed by patient's overall assessment, including hemodynamic status, amount of ongoing blood losses, and underlying comorbidities. Children with rapid loss of blood or associated major underlying comorbid condition such as congenital cyanotic heart disease or blood dyscrasias may even need blood transfusion at blood losses of <40% [6].

Although there can be no fixed numeric transfusion trigger in all trauma patients, few simple calculations can estimate allowable blood losses, which are:

Formula 1

$$Allowable\ Blood\ Loss(ABL) = \frac{\left[\begin{array}{l} \text{Estimated blood volume}(EBV) \times \\ (\text{Initial hematocrit} - \text{Target hematocrit}) \end{array} \right]}{\text{Hematocrit initial}}$$

Formula 2

$$Estimated\ Red\ Cell\ Mass(ERCM) = \text{Estimated blood volume}(EBV) \\ \times \text{Starting hematocrit}$$

$$Target\ Estimated\ Red\ Cell\ Mass(ERCM\ TARGET) = \text{Estimated blood volume}(EBV) \\ \times \text{Target hematocrit}$$

$$Allowable\ Red\ Cell\ Loss = ERCM - ERCM\ TARGET$$

$$ABL = ARCL \times 3$$

For replacement of allowable blood loss, in milliliters, it is multiplied by 3 if replaced with crystalloids and is replaced in 1:1 ratio if replaced by blood or colloid.

Nowadays in almost every center, blood banks provide individual components of blood-like packed cells, platelets, and plasma instead of complete blood as a measure to conserve resources and prevent unintentional wastage of blood products. Also it is more efficient and cost-effective measure by reducing transfusion of dispensible components and enabling components from a single blood donor accessible to several patients and preserves individual components.

9.4.2 Packed Red Blood Cells

Packed red cells are concentrated in 250 ml with hematocrit ranging between 60% and 80%. The preservative CDPA contains citrate which chelates calcium; hence calcium gluconate or calcium chloride must be given together with rapid blood transfusion to prevent severe hypocalcemia. PRBC are usually transfused in the dosage of *10–20 ml/kg*.

9.4.3 Fresh Frozen Plasma

Fresh frozen plasma (FFP) is thawed plasma containing several coagulation factors for hemostasis including labile factors like V and VIII and antithrombin III. Generally FFPs should be reserved in patients with abnormal blood test including deranged prothrombin time (PT) and activated partial thromboplastin time (APTT).

FFP is sometimes required in patients who receive >1 blood volume owing to nonsurgical bleeding (for immediate replacement of deficiencies of factors V and VIII). FFP is usually used in doses of 10–15 ml/kg.

9.4.4 Platelets

Massive blood transfusion can also result in dilution thrombocytopenia which further leads to nonsurgical or microvascular bleeding, and usually platelets have to be transfused before FFPs for this condition. 0.1 units/kg platelets is transfused to raise platelet count by approximately 20,000. More than 0.2 units/kg of platelet transfusion is rarely required as platelet count of 50,000 is usually sufficient for surgical hemostasis [7].

9.4.5 Cryoprecipitate

Cryoprecipitate is the insoluble portion of plasma which is produced by refreezing. This blood product has good content of factor VIII and fibrinogen. Hundred units of cryoprecipitate can be obtained from a single unit of FFP. The principal indications for transfusion of cryoprecipitate patients with trauma are disseminated intravascular coagulation (DIC), decreased fibrinogen levels, and other bleeding abnormalities after massive transfusion. The recommended dose of cryoprecipitate is 0.1 units/kg.

9.4.6   Massive Blood Replacement

Massive blood transfusion usually refers to the administration of one or more than one blood volume (approximately 75–80 ml/kg in children) within 24 h. It is associated with significant physiologic abnormalities like hypothermia, electrolyte, and acid-base abnormalities and coagulation defects. Following massive blood transfusion, there can be nonsurgical bleeding for which dilutional thrombocytopenia and clotting factor deficiencies are implicated. Therefore in children with ongoing blood loss and on massive transfusion (perioperative or preoperative), monitoring of coagulation profile is vital to prevent nonsurgical bleeding. The presence of acidosis, hypothermia, and hemodilution with hypofibrinogenemia may further exacerbate the coagulopathy. This perioperative evaluation can be easily performed by prothrombin time, partial thromboplastin time, and platelet count.

9.5   Monitoring and ICU Care

9.5.1   Cardiovascular

1. Electrocardiogram (ECG)
2. Noninvasive blood pressure (NIBP)
3. Vital signs at regular intervals
4. If patient is in shock and requires ionotropic support:
    (a) Continuous arterial blood pressure
    (b) Central venous pressure
    (c) Pulse pressure variation
    (d) Cardiac output monitoring (invasive and noninvasive)
    (e) SVR assessment
    (f) Echocardiography

9.5.2   Respiratory

1. Pulse oximetry
2. End tidal CO_2 monitoring
3. Ventilator alarms
4. Ventilator graphics

9.5.3   Central Nervous System

1. Monitoring of ICP (intracranial pressure) for head injury
2. Psychological/mental status evaluation (for prolonged ICU stay)

9.5.4   Auxiliary Monitors in ICU

(a) All patients with blood at urethral meatus must be assumed to have urethral injury as a consequence of pelvic trauma, and urinary catheterization should be done very gently in such patients.
(b) Retrograde urethrocystogram should be done to identify urethral injury in all cases who have abnormal findings on rectal examination or when one has a doubt on continuity of urethra.
(c) All patients with major abdominal trauma should have oral insertion of gastric drainage tube as the gastric dilatation may lead to significant impairment of respiration and hemodynamic compromise. Further management includes gastric decompression in such cases at earliest to decrease mortality. Apart from risk of aspiration, oral gastric tube also decreases the likelihood of sinusitis from obstruction of drainage pathways.

9.6   Pharmacology for Trauma in ICU

9.6.1   Volume Management

(a) Indications: findings or concerns for early shock or frank hypotension may be used to support hemodynamics while awaiting blood products in hemorrhagic shock.
(b) Initially give a 20 ml/kg IV bolus of crystalloids.
(c) Blood products: if no response to initial fluid bolus, give packed red blood cells (RBCs) 10 ml/kg IV [8].
(d) Advanced trauma life support (ATLS) principles must be followed for fluid replacement in the traumatized child (hemodynamically stable or unstable). It provides a good point of reference for the management of children with abdominal injuries (Fig. 9.1)

9.6.2   Analgesics

Pain in ICU patients can occur from various factors, such as preexisting trauma, invasive monitoring, and protracted serenity. Pain has often been neglected in patient under treatment in ICU setup especially in children. Traditionally it is feared

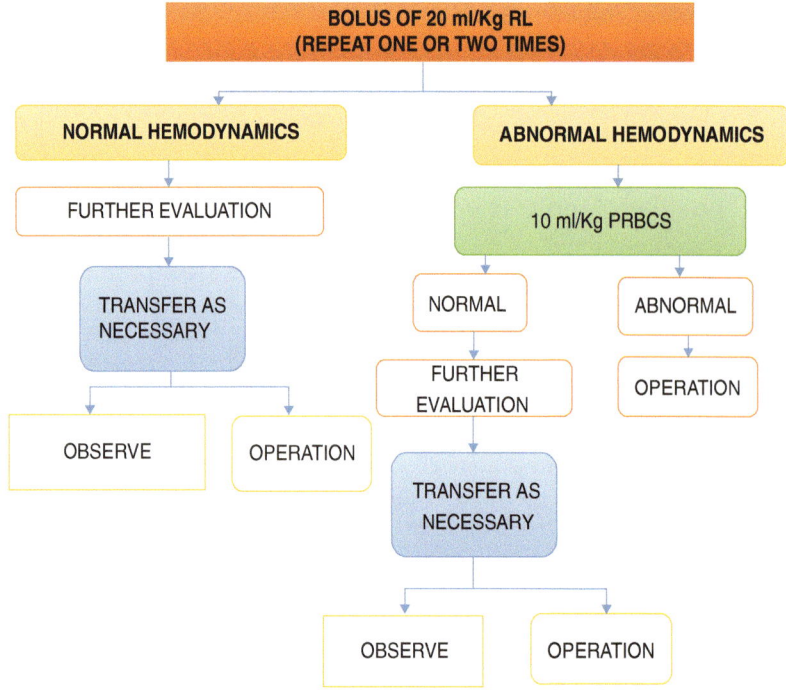

Fig. 9.1 Volume management algorithm for pediatric trauma patient

that opioids will mask symptoms of progressing injury. Various studies have however proven that the use of opioids does not result in significant masking of symptoms of the progressive disease.

Opioids are also feared for their unwarranted side effects like unexplained drowsiness and sometimes respiratory depression. These side effects can be evaded by using regional/local anesthesia techniques. Alleviation of pain in PICU setting should involve both non-pharmacological and pharmacological measures. Regional anesthesia involving simple intercostal nerve blocks, epidural analgesia, and paravertebral blocks are especially useful in children with rib fractures or flail chest [8, 9].

If a regional anesthesia cannot be instituted, a multimodal analgesic model of pain control using acetaminophen and NSAIDs can help reduce opioids required to treat pain. Under proper supervision, analgesia by patient-controlled mode (PCA) can be employed in children >5 years, with the provision to titrate opioid boluses as per their pain perception. Some commonly used drugs for analgesia in PICU are:

(a) Acetaminophen: 10–15 mg/kg orally four to six hourly; up to 75 mg/kg/day (effective for mild to moderate pain)
(b) Acetyl salicylic acid 30–65 mg/kg 4–6 h orally

(c) Codeine phosphate 3 mg/kg orally (contraindications—liver disease, ventilator failure, respiratory depression, head injury, excessive sedation)
(d) Diclofenac sodium 1–3 mg/kg 8 h (side effects: gastric bleed, ulceration)
(e) Ibuprofen—as antipyretic/analgesic 10–15 mg/kg 4–6 h
(f) Fentanyl: 1–2 µ/kg IV, if concern for unstable hemodynamics or early in resuscitation because of short-acting duration
(g) Morphine: 0.1 mg/kg IV; narcotic, gives superior analgesia and sedation

9.6.3 Anxiolytic/Sedatives

Sedation is a broad term when used in the context of PICU. It is usually employed for reducing awareness (from distressing ICU environment), to keep calm and restrained in a confined space, without interfering with monitors and IV lines. Different levels of sedation and anxiolysis may be required as per requirement for procedures like MRI/CT (deep sleep), physiotherapy (minor sedation), and adequate immobility for minor procedures (dressing, etc.). Different drugs fulfill these roles to varying extents [10]. Some commonly used drugs in PICU for sedation and anxiolysis are:

(a) Midazolam: provides sedation and anxiolytics; usually 0.1–0.2 mg/kg IV
(b) Promethazine (Phenergan): 0.1 mg/kg orally six hourly; max, 12.5 mg/dose during the day
(c) Propofol: 25–50 µ/kg/min drip, 0.5–1 mg/kg bolus
(d) Dexmedetomidine: provides adequate sedation and amnesia
    Initial dose: 1 µ/kg followed by maintenance dose of 0.2–0.7 µg/kg/h
(e) Lorazepam (for older children, >12 years of age)
    Initial dose: 2–3 mg orally (two to three times) per day
    Maintenance dose: 1–2 mg orally (two to three times) a day
(f) Triclofos sodium (Pedicloryl): 20 mg/kg orally

9.6.4 Muscle Relaxants

According to recent literature, the use of muscle relaxants should only be reserved in special circumstances. They are primarily used for intubation and for the procedures in which muscle relaxation is required so as to minimize the requirement of other anesthetic drugs. Atracurium and cisatracurium are preferred muscle relaxants in patients with liver and kidney injuries as they have Hoffman metabolism [10].

Some commonly used muscle relaxants in PICU are:

- Depolarizing
  - Suxamethonium: short-term neuromuscular blocker; 2 mg/kg IV; IM, double IV dose

- Nondepolarizing agents
  - Vecuronium: 0.1 mg/kg, 0.2 mg/kg if used for rapid sequence intubation
  - Cisatracurium: 0.1–0.15 mg/kg
  - Atracurium: bolus dose, 0.5 mg/kg; maintenance dose, 0.3–1.0 mg/kg/h
  - Rocuronium: bolus dose, 0.5 mg/kg; maintenance dose, 0.2–0.5 mg/kg/h

9.6.5 Inotropes and Other Drugs Frequently Used in PICU (as per Specific Case Requirement)

- Dobutamine: 3–20 mcg/kg/min
- Dopamine: 2–20 mcg/kg/min
- Norepinephrine: initial dose 0.05–0.1 mcg/kg/min, titrate to desired effect
- Furosemide: 0.5–1 mg/kg; max dose, 10 mg/kg/day
- Calcium gluconate
- Magnesium sulfate

9.7 Abdominal Compartment Syndrome in Blunt Trauma Abdomen

A sudden rise of intra-abdominal pressure over 20 mmHg as consequences of blunt trauma abdomen leading to multiple intra-abdominal organ failure or dysfunction due to compression effect leads to an entity, collectively known as abdominal compartment syndrome (ACS). This may or may not be associated with a decreased abdominal perfusion pressure (< 60 mmHg). It has a high mortality of more than 90%, if not timely deducted, and measures are taken to treat it on acute emergency basis. At most places, healthcare providers (especially dealing with pediatric patients) are not much familiar with the definition, monitoring, and treatment of ACS [11].

9.7.1 Measurement of IAP

Intra-abdominal pressure can be measured either directly or indirectly by various methods for diagnosis of ACS.

1. *Direct method*: In this method, a needle or catheter is placed in the abdominal cavity, and intra-abdominal pressure is measured by using a fluid column or pressure transducer system. It is considered as a gold standard method, but however it is not free of complications. The reported complications include bowel perforation, peritonitis, etc.
   (a) Direct method involves IAP measurement from the movement of a fluid column or pressure transducer system recorded via the catheter or a needle positioned into the peritoneal cavity.

2. *Indirect method*: It involves measurement of IAP from the pressure transmitted indirectly to the lumen of a hollow viscus intra-abdominal organ. Indirect measurements can be measured by using either intragastric, intra-rectal, intrauterine, venacaval, or intravesical methods.

   (a) Bladder method is the most accepted universally followed for indirect measurement. The pressure transducer is leveled at the cross section between lines joining iliac crests and the midaxillary line. Saline (in adequate amount) is infused into the bladder through a urinary catheter, and pressure is calculated once an equilibration with bladder pressure is reached. Although a minimum volume (03 ml) is recommended in children, a higher volume up to 25 ml (1 ml/kg) may be used to obtain an equilibrium IAP.

   Abdominal compartment syndrome (ACS) is further classified as:

1. Primary ACS is injury or disease directly originating from the abdomen or pelvis requiring surgery or interventional screening by radiologist.
2. Secondary ACS: ACS arises indirectly from conditions not originating primarily from the peritoneal cavity (abdomen) or pelvis.
3. Recurrent ACS: ACS redevelopment after previous successful treatment (medical/surgical or both) of ACS (primary or secondary).

9.7.2   Abdominal Compartment Syndrome (ACS): Treatment

Several options (surgical, medical, and interventional) are available for treatment of impending or existent intra-abdominal hypertension (IAH) (Table 9.1).

All available therapies should be utilized quickly for cases of continuing or increasing IAH. Decompression of the abdomen by surgical means (e.g., laparotomy) should be done and governed by patient's age and presence of organ dysfunction [12].

ACS can lead to a very high mortality to the range of 22–60% in children. If left unmanaged, multi-organ dysfunction ensues and is the major cause of high mortality in children. Therefore all steps should be taken to avoid point of no return, while cascade of inflammatory lesion ensues, and surgical decompression is no longer able to prevent impending mortality (incidence >90%).

9.8   Multi-organ Failure in Abdominal Compartment Syndrome: A Systemic Approach

A high mortality (22–60%) in children has been reported as the consequence of ACS secondary to multiple organ failure. This is because of increasing pressure effect from untreated ACS that can progress to multi-organ failure (MOF). Early intervention (especially surgical like laparotomy) may reduce the mortality in primary ACS patients by decreasing pressure and thus saving the underlying

Table 9.1 Tabulated account of options available for controlling intra-abdominal hypertension

Available options	Intraluminal content evacuation	Evacuation of intra-abdominal space-occupying lesions (SOL)	Abdominal wall compliance improvement	Fluid (IV) optimization	Optimization of perfusion pressure (both abdominal and systemic)
Medical options	Gastric/rectal tube Prokinetics Diet Fasting		Analgesics and sedatives Positioning Muscle relaxants	Modest fluid transfusion Diuretics	Goal-directed fluids Pressors Inotropes
Interventional (minimal invasive) options	Gastric and colonoscopic decompression	Paracentesis Catheter drainage (percutaneous)		Continuous venous hemofiltration	
Surgical (invasive options)		Decompressive laparotomy	Escharotomy or fasciotomy		Laparostomy (TAC)

TAC temporary abdominal closure (Adapted from Ejike et al. and Cheatham et al.)

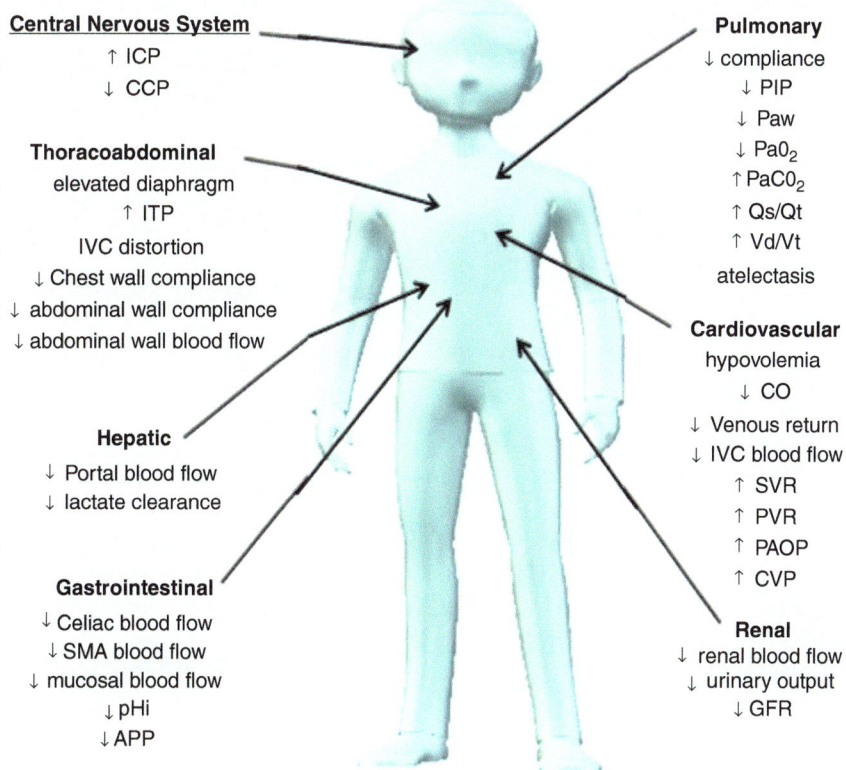

Central Nervous System
↑ ICP
↓ CCP

Thoracoabdominal
elevated diaphragm
↑ ITP
IVC distortion
↓ Chest wall compliance
↓ abdominal wall compliance
↓ abdominal wall blood flow

Hepatic
↓ Portal blood flow
↓ lactate clearance

Gastrointestinal
↓ Celiac blood flow
↓ SMA blood flow
↓ mucosal blood flow
↓ pHi
↓ APP

Pulmonary
↓ compliance
↓ PIP
↓ Paw
↓ PaO$_2$
↑ PaCO$_2$
↑ Qs/Qt
↑ Vd/Vt
atelectasis

Cardiovascular
hypovolemia
↓ CO
↓ Venous return
↓ IVC blood flow
↑ SVR
↑ PVR
↑ PAOP
↑ CVP

Renal
↓ renal blood flow
↓ urinary output
↓ GFR

Fig. 9.2 Diagrammatic representation of pathogenesis of multiple organ failure in abdominal compartment syndrome

intra-abdominal organs from impending failure. The multi-organ failure pathogenesis can be understood by following Fig. 9.2.

The major complication in blunt trauma abdomen patients is of concurrent inflammation and infection along with ACS resulting in multiple organ dysfunction (MODY) and failure. This MODY as the end result of uncontrolled ACS has a very high mortality rate (30–80%) despite best possible interventions.

9.8.1 Management of Multi-organ Failure

The main cornerstone of treatment in optimal management of multi-organ failure (MOF) with blunt trauma abdomen involves early recognition of IAH. Medical (nonsurgical) treatment should be tried first and at earliest with the goal of decreasing the intra-abdominal pressure by using one of these intervention methods:

- Gastric suctioning, rectal enemas, and sometimes prokinetic agents are used for evacuation of the intraluminal contents of the intestines.
- Paracentesis is often employed in evacuation of space-occupying abnormalities intra-abdominally or to correct extra-luminal pathological changes such as ascites, pneumoperitoneum, or hemoperitoneum.
- Goal-directed fluid therapy is required to optimize fluid administration; diuretics and continuous renal replacement therapy (CRRT) may be of paramount importance in decreasing overload of fluids and edema of the abdominal wall causing increased abdominal pressures.
- Adequate sedation, analgesia, and often muscle relaxation is required to improve abdominal wall compliance.
- A simple yet effective maneuver such as laying the patient supine can decrease IAP.

If the above nonoperative measures are not successful, then sometimes specific measures as surgical abdominal decompression by laparotomy may be required [13].

Not only abdominal compartment syndrome but solid abdominal organs such as the liver, kidney, lung, etc. may also undergo failure due to direct injury. In such cases, an organ-specific ICU care is needed which includes both conservative and often some sort of surgical intervention.

One should not forget that trauma victims are at risk of rhabdomyolysis due to crush injury and more so when reperfusion oxygenation of the limb is more than 6 h (warm ischemia time). Optimization of urine flow of approximately 1.5 ml/kg/h by vigorous expansion of plasma volume may lessen the degree of renal injury than those receiving late and lesser amounts of fluid therapy (https://www.ahcmedia.com/articles/138453-advances-in-pediatric-abdominal-trauma-whats-new-in-assessment-and-management).

9.9   Summary

Intensivists and anesthesiologists are the one called at first and have paramount role in managing pediatric cases with blunt trauma abdomen. They are not only required in resuscitation attempts but also play a critical role in the creation of trauma team. Trauma team is basically coordinated by a leader who not only follows a primary ABC of initial survey and resuscitation but is also involved in conducting a secondary survey and stabilization followed by prompt initiation and definite treatment. A thorough understanding of pathophysiology and special requirement of these population subsets helps in providing better care by exercising psychomotor skill, surgical judgment, and intellectual reasoning. A predetermined logistic approach for the management of the traumatized child with a meticulous plan of action not only guides to expeditious diagnosis and therapeutic intervention but also decreases the mortality. The role of anesthesiologists in care of such injured children is very vast ranging from admission to the casualty, surgical intervention, and postoperative care. Acquaintance with the different aspects of pediatric trauma allows anesthesia providers to be efficient and safe in their practice.

References

1. Nicol A, Steyn E. Oxford handbook of trauma for Southern Africa. Cape Town: Oxford University Press; 2004.
2. Nellensteijn DR. Pediatric abdominal injury: initial treatment and diagnostics. Groningen: Rijksuniversiteit Groningen; 2015.
3. Avarello JT, Cantor RM. Pediatric major trauma: an approach to evaluation and management. Emerg Med Clin North Am. 2007;25:803–36.
4. Wise BV, Mudd SS, Wilson ME. Management of blunt abdominal trauma in children. J Trauma Nurs. 2002;9(1):6–14.
5. Snehalata Dhayagude H, Nandini Dave M. Principles and practice of pediatric anesthesia. New Delhi: Jaypee Brothers Medical Publishers; 2016.
6. Bingham R, Thomas AL, Sury M. Hatch & Sumner's textbook of paediatric anaesthesia third edition. London: Edward Arnold; 2007.
7. Ivashkov Y, Bhananker SM. Perioperative management of pediatric trauma patients. Int J Crit Illn Inj Sci. 2012;2(3):143–8.
8. Cullen PM. Paediatric trauma. Contin Educ Anaesth Crit Care Pain. 2012;12(3):157–61.
9. Varon AJ, Smith CE, editors. Essentials of trauma anesthesia. Cambridge: Cambridge University Press; 2012.
10. Sutcliffe AJ. Paediatric trauma anaesthesia. Curr Anaesth Crit Care. 1996;7(3):146–51.
11. Kaussen T, Steinau G, Srinivasan PK, et al. Recognition and management of abdominal compartment syndrome among German pediatric intensivists. Ann Intensive Care. 2012;2(Suppl 1):S8.
12. Schacherer N, Miller J, Petronis K. Pediatric blunt abdominal trauma in the emergency department: evidence-based management techniques. Pediatr Emerg Med Pract. 2014;11:1–23.
13. McFadyen JG, Ramaiah R, Bhananker SM. Initial assessment and management of pediatric trauma patients. Int J Crit Illn Inj Sci. 2012;2(3):121–7.

Blunt Solid Organ Injuries in Children

10

Rizwan Ahmad Khan

It is reported that the incidence of solid organ injuries in children with blunt abdominal trauma varies from 4% to 8% depending on the site of injury and the mode of impact. Most cases of solid organ injuries in children are minor grade, with only few injuries involving major parenchymal or vascular disruptions. The optimal management of pediatric patients with solid organ injury has shifted toward nonoperative management. But the management of high-grade injuries remains poorly defined and relies heavily on associated factors. This paradigm shift in treatment protocol of solid organ injury has many advantages. It means reducing the hospital stay and cost and less operative and postoperative complications for patients. It also means management "at home" or with the primary care pediatrician, thereby allowing intensivist and pediatric surgeon to allocate ample amount of time to more critical cases. Since children are usually healthy, with not many comorbid conditions and hardly on any medications, they are able to withstand the hemodynamic instability much better than adults [1].

10.1 Pancreas

Although pancreatic injury is not so common in children it still accounts for 3–12% incidence following blunt trauma to abdomen. However the morbidity associated with pancreatic injury is highest among the solid organs. The mortality is mostly related to the associated injury. The retroperitoneal position of the pancreas often results in a characteristic late presentation of symptoms. Therefore, following blunt trauma to the abdomen, signs of pancreatic injury should be specifically looked for to prevent high morbidity associated with late detection of pancreatic injury [2]. Pancreatic injury should be suspected based on the history of upper abdominal

R. A. Khan
Department of Pediatric Surgery, Jawaharlal Nehru Medical College, AMU,
Aligarh, Uttar Pradesh, India

© Springer Nature Singapore Pte Ltd. 2018
R. Ahmad Khan, S. Wahab (eds.), *Blunt Abdominal Trauma in Children*,
https://doi.org/10.1007/978-981-13-0692-1_10

injury or presence of visible upper abdominal ecchymoses. The clinical examination may not reveal any abnormality in initial hours. Therefore it is advisable to regularly reassess the patients of suspected pancreatic injury. Another compounding problem is that the laboratory investigations and radiologic imaging modalities may be sensitive but not specific or characteristic for only pancreatic injuries. The serum amylase level cannot always be relied as an indicator for pancreatic injury since it is frequently not initially raised after the injury. Therefore, a repeated assessment of serum amylase is recommended. Similarly neither initial nor the peak values of serum amylase/lipase have been shown to have any analytical efficacy for predicting the grade of pancreatic injury. The sensitivity of ultrasound varies significantly depending upon the hemodynamic status of patient and technical expertise and thus has a low accuracy for diagnosing pancreatic injury. CT provides better delineation of and location of parenchymal lesions. CT scan has increased accuracy in imaging pancreatic lesions. For detailed role of imaging, refer to chapter on imaging. To evaluate the pancreatic duct and its integrity, magnetic resonance cholangiopancreatography (MRCP) and endoscopic retrograde cholangiopancreatography (ERCP) are the preferred imaging modalities. However, experience with these techniques in injuries of pancreas in pediatric age group is very restricted. It is also an invasive procedure with significant complications especially in smaller children. Table 10.1 shows the grading of pancreatic injury by AAST.

For most of the minor grade injuries of the solid organs in children, nonoperative management has become the standard of care. However there are considerable controversy and disagreement over the treatment and timing of high-grade injuries [3].

10.1.1 Grade I and II Injuries

If there are no associated injuries which require operative intervention, grade I and II pancreatic injuries are generally managed conservatively. This involves withholding enteral nutrition and total parenteral nutrition and nasogastric drainage for associated ileus. The use of proton pump inhibitors and perhaps octreotide is also recommended. Although in practice most of the surgeons use proton pump inhibitors or octreotide, there has been no conclusive studies on the benefits of these agents. Some authors advocate simple external drainage for managing small

Table 10.1 AAST grading of pancreatic injury

Grade	Type of injury	Description of injury
I	Hematoma	Minor contusion without duct injury
	Laceration	Superficial laceration without duct injury
II	Hematoma	Major contusion without duct injury or tissue loss
	Laceration	Major laceration without duct injury or tissue loss
III	Laceration	Distal transection or parenchymal injury with duct injury
IV	Laceration	Proximal transection involving ampulla
V	Laceration	Massive disruption of pancreatic head

lacerations or contusions with the rationale that drainage of activated proteolytic enzymes decreases the risk of complication of pancreatic injury, e.g., pancreatic abscess, pancreatic fistulae, and pseudocysts. However, a recent retrospective study on more than 100 children with minor grade pancreatic injuries concluded that the rate of recovery and resolution of pancreatic injury with nonoperative management were good and comparable with surgical treatment [4]. No significant difference in outcome between the children with class I injuries who managed nonoperatively and those who underwent surgical treatment was seen.

10.1.2 Grade III and IV Injuries

The frequency of the occurrence of high-grade pancreatic or ductal injury following blunt abdominal trauma is quite low 0.12% [4, 5].

The management of grade III injuries involving transection of distal body or pancreatic parenchyma injury involving the main pancreatic duct is both variable and controversial. A nonoperative approach is promoted by those authors who maintain that subsequent development of traumatic pseudocysts can be managed with or without percutaneous drainage or by internal pseudocyst drainage (open or endoscopic drainage into stomach or bowel, mostly jejunum). Other surgeons favor spleen-sparing distal pancreatectomy for grade III injuries since this has the advantage of being a definite surgical procedure associated with a quick recovery and the morbidity associated with development and maturity of pseudocyst is also greatly reduced. Some advocate expectant treatment leading to formation of pseudocyst which can be later managed by drainage procedure. Other options include suturing the stump and distal Roux-en-Y pancreatojejunostomy or repair of primary duct with drainage. Lately endoscopic management is advocated which involves ERCP and stenting. High-grade pancreatic injury involving the pancreatic head (grade IV injury) can be treated conservatively initially, thereby allowing the formation of pseudocysts which can be managed easily by drainage procedure. Most of the authors advocate aggressive management in early detected grade IV injury by Roux-en-Y jejunal onlay, pylorus-preserving pancreatoduodenectomy [4].

10.1.3 Delayed Detected Injuries

There are many anecdotal cases reported in literature regarding management of late detected injuries. Delayed detection of proximal ductal transection can be treated by wide surgical drainage without pancreatic resection. In follow-up there are reports of spontaneous recanalization, or if pseudocyst develops, then it can be managed with drainage procedure later on. Simple drainage supplemented with sphincterotomy may also help heal proximal duct injuries.

Another approach promoted is ERCP to determine the precise diagnosis and the assessment of the extent of injury to parenchyma or main duct of pancreas in addition to endonasal pancreatic drainage (ENPD) followed by primary anastomosis and repair of the damaged duct. A short-term TPN may help the healing [5].

10.1.4 Failure of Nonoperative Management

The failure of NOM occurs in cases where there is high-grade pancreatic injury and patient have multiple pancreatic injuries. The patient characteristics are multiple intra-abdominal injuries and those with a higher grade of pancreatic injury. It has been reported that timely transfer to pediatric trauma center has been associated with less failure of nonoperative management. Children with significantly higher Injury Severity Score are also at risk of failed nonoperative management. Nonresponding hemodynamic instability is another guide for failure of nonoperative management. Radiographic evidence of ongoing hemorrhage known as "contrast blush" indicating contrast extravasation has been associated with failed conservative management. Most of the children who do not improve with conservative management fail initially in the course of the treatment. The peak failure rate is at 4 h following admission and initiation of the conservative treatment. Therefore it is recommended that the child must undergo regular and continuous surgical evaluation right from admission, through stabilization and discharge.

10.1.5 Role of ERCP

Endoscopic retrograde cholangiopancreatography (ERCP) is the modality of choice for diagnosing ductal injury. It has an added advantage of allowing therapeutic intervention as well in the patients of pancreatic injury.

ERCP is fairly safe in pediatric age group particularly if the performing surgeon has good expertise with children and some authors recommend using ERCP routinely in patients with significant pancreatic injury. ERCP is a valuable screening procedure which identifies ductal injury with accuracy and accordingly makes possible deciding whether conservative management or operative intervention is required. It offers an additional benefit of allowing intervening like placement of stent in children with main duct transection. Although ERCP may help avoid pancreatic resection, it does not safeguard against development of pseudocyst or pancreatic fluid collections requiring drainage [6, 7].

10.1.6 Pseudocyst

Pseudocyst formation is the most frequently observed complication following pancreatic trauma which has been managed conservatively. Pseudocyst formation is supposed to be due to the higher grades of pancreatic injury involving the duct as well (grade III or IV injury). It is described to occur in up to 10% of children sustaining high-grade injuries. The frequency of formation of pseudocyst is high, but there is high rate of resolution on its own, and the rest can be managed easily with drainage procedures. The level of serum amylase more than 1100 U/L is said to be predictive for developing a pseudocyst. For small and immature pseudocyst, conservative management is advised which includes bowel rest and total parental nutrition. This heals most of the pseudocyst in the majority of these children. Larger and mature pseudocysts that fail to resolve conservatively over time or those with complications like infection or bowel obstruction may be treated by percutaneous drainage. Most of these persistent posttraumatic pseudocysts are however amenable to internal enteric drainage. However some may require major interventions in the form of distal pancreatic resections or drainage procedures for pancreatic fistula. The development of a pseudocyst is considered to be a physiologic healing mechanism of the body after severe pancreatic injury, and it should be taken as a positive outcome rather than as a complication since its management is easy and definite [8].

10.2   Spleen

The most common solid organ to be injured in children sustaining blunt trauma to abdomen is spleen. Blunt splenic injury is usually associated with high-energy motor vehicle accidents causing sudden compression of the abdominal or thoracic wall. There has been a paradigm shift in treatment protocol of blunt splenic injury in children with a trend toward nonoperative management which responds in more than 90% of the cases across most injury grades (grades I–IV) Table 10.2. Even in children with grade V injury (Fig. 10.1), more than 30% can be managed nonoperatively. The American Pediatric Surgical Association has given evidence-based guidelines for the management of patients with stable hemodynamic parameters with isolated liver or spleen injuries. These guidelines were laid down keeping in view the optimum utilization of resources and to set a standard for admission and monitoring in the intensive care unit (ICU), indications for radiological imaging, and the total length of admission in the hospital. The children with low-grade injuries and stable hemodynamic parameters should be admitted and monitored in general wards, thereby avoiding needless expenditure that usually occurs with intensive care unit monitoring. It also advocated that the follow-up imaging should only be reserved for high-grade injuries (grades III, IV, and V) that have been managed conservatively, to document proper healing before allowing the child to return to unmonitored activity [9, 10].

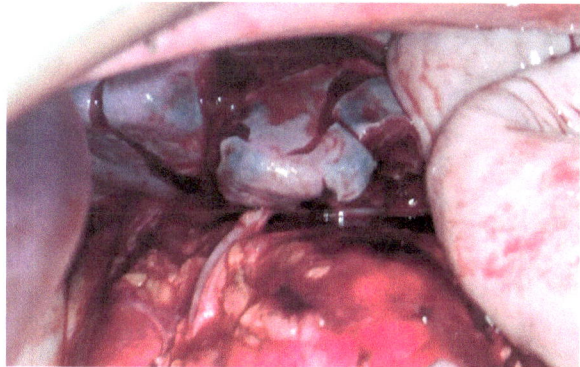

Fig. 10.1 Shattered spleen in a child with blunt abdominal trauma

Table 10.2 AAST grading of splenic injury

Grade	Type of injury	Description of injury
I	Hematoma	Subcapsular, <10% surface area
	Laceration	<1 cm parenchymal depth
II	Hematoma	Subcapsular, 10–50% surface area; intraparenchymal, <5 cm
	Laceration	1–3 cm parenchymal depth
III	Hematoma	Subcapsular, >50% surface area; intraparenchymal, >5 cm
	Laceration	>3 cm parenchymal depth
IV	Laceration	Segmental or hilar vessels; 4 devascularization >25% spleen
V	Laceration	Completely shattered spleen
	Vascular	Hilar injury with splenic devascularization

Various operative and interventional radiological procedures are advised for children who fail nonoperative management. Spleen-preserving procedures like splenorrhaphy and partial splenectomy have been reported by some authors to preserve splenic tissue, but it has been seen that majority of these patients ultimately lose their spleen. Radiographic embolization is another technique that may help prevent splenectomy [11, 12]. Children who require splenectomy should receive vaccination against *Streptococcus pneumoniae*, *Haemophilus influenzae* type b, and *Neisseria meningitides* along with oral penicillin chemoprophylaxis.

10.3 Liver

Blunt injury to the liver is the second most common injury to solid intra-abdominal organ following blunt abdominal injury in children. Contrary to splenic trauma, blunt injury to the liver carries significant mortality especially high-grade injuries. However, a success rate of more than 90% in blunt liver trauma in children and decreased rate of morbidity, transfusions, and complications have made the nonoperative management the first choice among most pediatric surgeons. Children who have sustained blunt liver injury and are stabilized using fluid resuscitation alone are more likely to respond to nonoperative management. There is poor correlation between the grade of hepatic injury as assessed by CT scan and the need for surgical intervention. The CT scan findings alone cannot guide the operative intervention in a hemodynamically stable child, but regular clinical examination and a high index of suspicion for potential failure must be kept in mind to avoid poor outcome with delayed intervention [13].

The indications for emergency surgery following hepatic injury in children include unstable hemodynamic parameters, evidence of continuing bleeding, and presence of other associated injuries like bowel injury or pancreatic injury. Hemodynamic instability in hepatic injury is defined as a requirement of transfusions of more than 25 mL/kg within the initial 2 h of presentation.

Most low-grade hepatic injuries necessitating operative intervention can be managed by simple methods of hemostasis like manual compression, hepatorrhaphy, suture ligation of bleeding vessel, and topical hemostatic agents. However management of unstable and nonresponsive patients becomes a challenge if critical physiologic and metabolic consequences start to develop. These include prolonged operations with massive blood product replacement and resultant development of hypothermia, coagulopathy, and acidosis. This lethal triad generates a vicious cycle in which one complication supplements the other, thereby leading to uncontrolled pathophysiology. It is in these cases that "damage control surgery" is indicated wherein the approach is packing for hemostasis, permitting resuscitation in ICU setup and then again reexploring with a definite plan. "Damage control" treatment strategy is a structured and gradual approach in the surgical treatment of the bleeding trauma patient. Continued falling physiologic parameters and anatomic difficulty are the usual triggers for switching to damage control during laparotomy. These include intraoperative pH <7.2, core temperature <35 °C, and prothrombin time >16 s. Surgically it involves perihepatic packing and temporary abdominal closure followed by monitoring in ICU. The parameters that need to be optimized are urine output, mixed venous and arterial oxygen saturation, serum lactate, and base deficit. The patients are rewarmed, oxygen delivery is optimized, and coagulation factors are replaced. This can be supplemented with interventional imaging measures like angiographic embolization, and endoscopic stenting of damaged biliary tree may be required for controlling bleeding or for planning surgical approach. The next phase involves returning to the operation theater for relook and removal of packs and definitive management of injuries. However, packing may be associated with major morbidity such as intra-abdominal sepsis and risk of abdominal compartment syndrome and resultant organ failure. To prevent abdominal compartment syndrome, temporary abdominal wall closure at the initial surgery is advocated.

The success of the abridged laparotomy and planned reoperation lies in the critical balance between the timely institution of all the phases of damage control strategy and availability of advanced surgical care and surgical proficiency [14].

Delayed complications following hepatic injury include hemorrhage, bile leaks, hemobilia, infections, and pseudoaneurysms. Most of these can be easily managed by conservative and interventional imaging and endoscopic techniques. Angiographic embolization has proven effective for patients with continued hemorrhage or hemobilia. Image-guided percutaneous drainage and endoscopic internal stenting are routinely employed for the treatment of bilomas and bile duct injuries [15] (Table 10.3).

Table 10.3 AAST grade for hepatic injury

Grade	Type of injury	Description of injury
I	Hematoma	Subcapsular, <10% surface area
	Laceration	<1 cm parenchymal depth
II	Hematoma	Subcapsular, 10–50% surface area; intraparenchymal, <10 cm
	Laceration	1–3 cm parenchymal depth <10 cm length
III	Hematoma	Subcapsular, >50% surface area; intraparenchymal, >10 cm
	Laceration	>3 cm parenchymal depth
IV	Laceration	Laceration disruption of 25–75% of lobe
V	Laceration	Disruption of >75% of lobe
	Vascular	Juxtahepatiic venous injury
VI	Vascular	Hepatic avulsion

References

1. Keller MS. Blunt injury to solid abdominal organs. Semin Pediatr Surg. 2004;13:106–11.
2. Mattix KD, Tataria M, Holmes J, et al. Pediatric pancreatic trauma: predictors of nonoperative management failure and associated outcomes. J Pediatr Surg. 2007;42:340–4.
3. Lutz N, Mahboubi S, Nance ML, Stafford PW. The significance of contrast blush on computed tomography in children with splenic injuries. J Pediatr Surg. 2004;39:491–4.
4. Partrick DA, Bensard DD, Moore EE, Karrer FM. Nonoperative management of solid organ injuries in children results in decreased blood utilization. J Pediatr Surg. 1999;34:1695–9.
5. Nance ML, Lutz N, Carr MC, et al. Blunt renal injuries in children can be managed nonoperatively: outcome in a consecutive series of patients. J Trauma. 2004;57:474–8.
6. Fulcher AS, Turner MA, Yelon JA, et al. Magnetic resonance cholangiopancreatography (MRCP) in the assessment of pancreatic duct trauma and its sequelae: preliminary findings. J Trauma. 2000;48:1001–7.
7. Tepas JJ 3rd, Frykberg ER, Schinco MA, et al. Pediatric trauma is very much a surgical disease. Ann Surg. 2003;237:775–80.
8. Holmes JH 4th, Tataria M, Mattix KD, et al. The failure of nonoperative management in solid organ injury: a multi-institutional pediatric trauma center experience. J Trauma. 2005;59:1309–13.
9. Puapong D, Brown CV, Katz M, et al. Angiography and the pediatric trauma patient: a 10-year review. J Pediatr Surg. 2006;41:1859–63.
10. De Jong WJJ, Nellensteijn DR, ten Duis HJ, Albers MJIJ, El Moumni M, Hulscher JBF. Blunt splenic trauma in children: are we too careful? Eur J Pediatr Surg. 2011;21(4):234–7.
11. Feliciano PD, Mullins RJ, Trunkey DD, Crass RA, Beck JR, Helfand M. A decision analysis of traumatic splenic injuries. J Trauma. 1992;33:340–7.
12. Davis DH, Localio AR, Stafford PW, et al. Trends in operative management of pediatric splenic injury in a regional trauma system. Pediatrics. 2005;115:89–94.
13. Landau A, van As AB, Numanoglu A, Millar AJW, Rode H. Liver injuries in children: the role of selective non-operative management. Injury. 2006;37:66–71.
14. van der Vlies CH, Saltzherr TP, Wilde JC, van Delden OM, de Haan RJ, Goslings JC. The failure rate of nonoperative management in children with splenic or liver injury with contrast blush on computed tomography: a systematic review. J Pediatr Surg. 2010;45(5):1044–9.
15. Giss SR, Dobrilovic N, Brown RL, Garcia VF. Complications of nonoperative management of pediatric blunt hepatic injury: diagnosis, management, and outcomes. J Trauma. 2006;61(2):334–9.

Genitourinary Injuries in Pediatric Blunt Trauma

11

Tanveer Roshan Khan and Rizwan Ahmad Khan

11.1 Introduction

Traumatic injury, intentional or unintentional, is the main cause of deaths in children and adolescents than all other causes put together. Blunt form of trauma is a more common injury in children. The penetrating type of trauma constitutes 10–20% of all admissions in children with the increase in violence among 13–18-year-olds. It must be stressed that the pediatric patient is different physiologically from an adult counterpart but the basic principles remain the same [1].

Injuries to genitourinary system in children are important because management has a significant impact on future sexual health and therefore the psychological development of the child. The diverse nature of the cause and effect of these injuries in children makes it a difficult task for the attending pediatric surgeon. The injuries can range from simple contact dermatitis of the external genital organs to major renal trauma [2].

Genitourinary (GU) injuries in children are mostly associated with polytrauma; thoracic, head, and other abdominal injuries are commonly associated with GU injuries in children. As for other injuries, the attending pediatric surgeon must prioritize the injuries so that the precise management plan can be implemented.

As far as the prevention of these injuries is concerned, educational programs and guidelines must be implemented which should focus on decreasing the occurrence of GU injuries in children.

T. R. Khan (✉)
Department of Pediatric Surgery, RML, Lucknow, Uttar Pradesh, India

R. A. Khan
Department of Pediatric Surgery, Jawaharlal Nehru Medical College, AMU, Aligarh, Uttar Pradesh, India

© Springer Nature Singapore Pte Ltd. 2018
R. Ahmad Khan, S. Wahab (eds.), *Blunt Abdominal Trauma in Children*,
https://doi.org/10.1007/978-981-13-0692-1_11

Due to children's weaker abdominal muscles, less ossified and protective rib cage, paucity of perirenal fat, intra-abdominal renal location, and relatively larger kidney-to-body size ratio, they have a greater risk of blunt kidney injury. Approximately 10% of children presenting with blunt trauma to the abdomen have injury related to the kidney [1, 2].

11.2   Renal Injuries

The most common organ of the urogenital system to be injured in children is the kidney. The basis for this is the size (large for body) and its lower position in the retroperitoneum. This together with the absence of well-developed Gerota's fascia and pliability of the 11th and 12th ribs in children makes them susceptible to injury. The associated anomalies like hydronephrosis or tumor also makes it susceptible to trauma [2].

11.2.1 Mechanism

The mechanism which is most commonly postulated for the renal injury in blunt trauma is the abrupt deceleration forces which lead to crushing of kidneys against the vertebral column or the ribs. This usually leads to contusion and laceration of the kidneys. These deceleration injuries can also cause stretching of renal vessels in the relatively fixed vascular pedicle. The most commonly seen mode of deceleration injuries is fall and sports-related injuries. The direct injuries due to penetrating objects of fractured bony fragments can disrupt the renal parenchyma and collecting system.

11.2.2 Clinical Features

History of injury to flank by direct blow or motor vehicle accidents suggestive of considerable deceleration forces should raise the suspicion of renal injury. While the presence of ecchymosis or tenderness in flank region is also suggestive of renal injury, in a quarter of all the cases of blunt renal injury, there is no clinical sign or symptom suggesting renal injury. The presence of tenderness is an important sign in evaluating a blunt abdominal trauma patient, but it may not be present in half the children with significant blunt renal injury.

Inspection of perineum may give significant clues to genitourinary trauma, e.g., the presence of perineal ecchymosis, swelling, laceration, bleeding, etc. are quite indicative of some genitourinary involvement. Digital rectal examination is of utmost importance in evaluating these children. A high-riding prostate is highly suggestive of severe urethral injury, and before attempting urethral cannulation, a formal urethrography is advised. The presence of blood at the urinary meatus or a gross hematuria is suggestive of renal trauma and requires further urological imaging. If an X-ray of KUB reveals the presence of a pelvic fracture with associated hematuria, then bladder involvement must be suspected. This can be confirmed with cystography. A widened symphysis pubis and fractures of the sacrum are strong predictors of bladder injury [3], while fracture of inferior pubic ramus indicates urethral injuries. Thus hematuria is an important sign of renal injury even in microscopic form. However, the absence of hematuria does not rule out the involvement of the kidneys and the tracts.

11.2.3 Evaluation

The good radiological evaluation is key to successful management of urinary tract injuries. A child who is presenting with suspected renal injury and any amount of hematuria should be subjected to radiographic evaluation of the urinary tracts. Ultrasound is extensively used in evaluating blunt abdominal trauma. However, it can only evaluate the presence of free fluid in the peritoneal cavity and focuses on major solid organs intraperitoneally. Ultrasound is not a sensitive modality for detecting renal parenchymal injuries. However in expert hands and with application of Doppler, even vascular injuries can be diagnosed correctly. Overall the utility of ultrasound in acute phase is limited [4]. In children with associated head injury, however, it can rapidly rule out intraperitoneal blood. Computed tomography is the investigation of choice in evaluating hemodynamically stable patient. The nonionic contrast is used in the dosage of 2–3 mL/kg. The CT scan can give the clear-cut delineation of parenchymal injuries, functional status of the kidneys, any extravasation, or any pedicle injuries [5].

11.2.4 Grading

The grading of renal injuries is given by AAST (Table 11.1).

Table 11.1 The AAST grading for renal injuries

Grade	Type of injury	Description of injury
I	Contusion	Microscopic or gross hematuria
	Hematoma	Subcapsular nonexpanding without parenchymal laceration
II	Hematoma	Nonexpanding perirenal hematoma confined to renal retroperitoneum
	Laceration	<1 cm parenchymal depth of renal cortex without urinary extravasation
III	Laceration	>1 cm parenchymal depth of renal cortex without urinary extravasation
IV	Laceration	Laceration extending through the cortex, medulla, and collecting system
	Vascular	Main renal artery or vein injury with contained hemorrhage
V	Laceration	Completely shattered kidney
	Vascular	Main vessel avulsion injury with devascularization of the kidney

11.2.5 Management

In hemodynamically stable children suffering with high-grade renal injury (AAST grades IV–V), the nonoperative management is safe and reliable and has become the standard care. It has been revealed by many authors that even if the delayed intervention is required in these patients, it has not increased nephrectomy rates. Therefore it is recommended that retroperitoneal exploration should not be attempted in children with hemodynamically stable renal injuries [4].

Some authors who favor immediate surgical intervention in these children argue that there are unreliable clinical predictors of shock in children: high nephrectomy rates and the risk of severe hypertension as reasons with delayed intervention. But these risks are not proven. Other rare complications of nonoperative management are urinoma, fever, ileus, and pain. The use of minimally invasive techniques (endourologic and embolization) is helpful in management of acute phase and complications. When available, they help control the hemorrhage and decrease chances of renal loss. Arteriography with selective embolization for severe bleeding (requiring more than two transfusions) may be tried before exploring the injury. For localized unresolving hematoma/urinoma, percutaneous drainage is the procedure of choice [6].

11.2.6 Renovascular Injuries

Major renal pedicle injuries are rarely seen in children. The mechanism for renal pedicle injury is supposed to be rapid deceleration forces which cause stretching of the vessels resulting in varying grades of vascular trauma. Even if complete or partial avulsion is not present, the minor form of injuries may cause injury to the arterial intima and resultant arterial thrombosis. The blunt renal vascular injuries are more common on the left side since it is close to the aorta and shorter in length and therefore cannot endure the stretching force affected by deceleration.

The signs of renal pedicle injury on CECT are (1) the absence of renal enhancement, (2) central hematoma, (3) sudden cutoff in an enhanced renal artery, and (4) non-enhancement of the pelvicaliceal system.

The management depends on presentation, grade of the vessel involvement, and the extent of injury to the renal and other retroperitoneal structures. The primary repair is easier on the left side as compare to the right side. The left-sided renal vein avulsion injury at its origin can be handled by simple ligation due to the fact that gonadal and adrenal veins usually allow adequate collateral drainage [6].

11.2.7 Complications

However the nonoperative management of renal injuries leads to high rate of complications. The patients on nonoperative management should be closely monitored perhaps in an ICU setting. Any indicator of continued bleeding like falling hematocrit, continuous transfusion requirements, and presence of hematuria should warrant immediate intervention. It must be evaluated with a repeat CT scan or arteriogram. If interventional imaging facility is available, then selective embolization is the procedure of choice to localize and control the bleeding. Otherwise or in the presence of continuous bleeding not amenable to interventional imaging, procedure must be taken for emergent operative exploration. Incidence of delayed episodes of renal bleeding is rare and rarely reported beyond 2 weeks of injury. The arteriovenous fistula and pseudoaneurysm related to renal vascular injuries may be effectively treated by percutaneous endovascular embolization. Persistent urinary extravasation or urinoma presents with prolonged ileus, fever, and abdominal/flank mass. Most of the small non-infected urinomas in children do not require any intervention as they resolve on their own. However large and infected collections require percutaneous drainage or endoscopic placement of ureteral stents with broad-spectrum antibiotic coverage. Other late complications may include renal hypertension and hydronephrosis stone disease [7].

11.2.8 Follow-Up/Outcomes

Abdalati et al. suggested a follow-up protocol of children with renal injury. Since grades I and II injuries heal completely, they required only clinical follow-up. The grade III injuries have the highest rate of complications (30%). Therefore grade III injuries are to be followed by CT, scintigraphy, and/or ultrasound for every 3–4 months until complete healing is demonstrated. Grade IV injuries also require radiologic follow-up to evaluate complications and renal function. For assessment of renal function scintigraphy, using quantitative dimercaptosuccinic acid (DMSA) is a more useful than CT scan which allows anatomic details [8].

11.3 Ureteral Trauma

The ureteral injury is rare in children and constitutes only 1% of all urologic traumas. There are high chances of ureteropelvic junction disruption in children as the kidneys are relatively placed low against a pliable ribcage making them susceptible to stretching forces. Almost all ureteral injuries are associated with other injuries. Clinical suspicion combined with CT enhances the chance of early detection of ureteral injuries. The goal of the treatment is to restore the continuity so as to maintain the renal function. According to the nature of injury, the commonly done procedures are ureteroneocystostomy, ureteroureterostomy, autotransplant, transureteroureterostomy, Boari flap, etc. All these procedures must be done in elective setting in a hemodynamically stabilized patient and not in emergent setup. The procedures can be done by endoscopic, surgical, or a combination of both [9, 10].

11.4   Bladder Injuries

Although the bladder injuries in children are uncommon, the blunt bladder injuries predominate all types of bladder injuries. The most common mode is the direct blow to the lower abdomen in a distended bladder. Another mode is shearing force on bladder from the fascial attachments following pelvic fracture or direct laceration from pelvic fracture. Road traffic accidents involving motor vehicle accidents are the most common followed by fall from height and direct blow injuries [11, 12].

11.4.1 Classification

The two types of bladder injury encountered are contusion and ruptures. A contusion of bladder involves the disruptions of the muscular layer only, and the epithelial wall is intact. They do not require any surgical intervention and heal spontaneously. Bladder rupture, complete disruption of the bladder wall, is further classified as extraperitoneal and intraperitoneal ruptures. Extraperitoneal bladder ruptures are more common (60–65%), while intraperitoneal ruptures occur in one-fourth of cases; the combined injury is seen in 10–15% of cases. A pelvic fracture injury is more frequently associated with extraperitoneal bladder rupture, but it can cause intraperitoneal rupture also. The most common site for intraperitoneal rupture is the dome of the bladder. It must be kept in mind that in infants and young children, the bladder is an intraperitoneal organ and any bladder injury will lead to intraperitoneal extravasation of urine [12].

11.4.2 Management

11.4.2.1   Bladder Contusions
Almost all bladder contusions are managed nonoperatively. They heal without any sequelae. However, in patients having associated large pelvic hematoma, temporary per urethral catheter drainage is required.

11.4.2.2   Intraperitoneal Rupture
The most common site for intraperitoneal rupture is the dome of the bladder which is also the weakest and most mobile part of the bladder. Intraperitoneal rupture is more common in children. This form of bladder rupture is often associated with other major injuries, entailing a detailed urological workup. Since prolonged extravasation of urine into the peritoneal cavity can lead to severe metabolic and septic complications, early operative intervention for intraperitoneal bladder rupture is indicated. Most of the delayed presenting patients have severely deranged renal functions, and biochemical profile is akin to acute renal failure patient. The bladder is accessed through a lower midline abdominal incision. Intraperitoneal bladder injuries at the dome are repaired in two layers with absorbable suture. In the postoperative period, transurethral catheter drainage is done. The bladder rent may be

widened to inspect the bladder inside. The associated extraperitoneal ruptures can be repaired from inside the bladder in single running layer with an absorbable suture. During bladder repair, care must be given to localization of ureters, and any injuries near bladder neck must be repaired with great care so as to avoid any urinary incontinence [13, 14].

11.4.2.3 Extraperitoneal Rupture

If the diagnosis of an extraperitoneal rupture is made preoperatively by contrast extravasation, then the ideal management is per urethral catheter drainage alone. With per urethral drainage, most of the ruptures tend to heal within 10 days, while rest may take up to 3 weeks making it as safe and effective treatment modality of extraperitoneal rupture. This avoids unnecessary bladder exploration which has more complications.

If extraperitoneal rupture needs to be repaired, it should be done via an intravesical approach. It is repaired in a single running layer of an absorbable suture with catheter drainage of bladder [14, 15].

11.5 Urethral Injuries

Blunt abdominal trauma leading to pelvic fracture is the most common setting for a posterior urethral injury in a child. However, only 5% of children with pelvic fracture will have an injury to the posterior urethra. Among them 10–20% are coupled with bladder injury. Ninety percent of urethral injuries are due to motor vehicle accidents. The other modes of injury are fall from height, sports, and crush injuries [15].

The mechanism for anterior urethral injuries is straddle injuries. The diagnosis of injury to urethra is usually straightforward. The symptoms indicative of urethral injury are inability to void, blood at meatus, and gross hematuria. The clinical examination of the genitals and the perineum may show the presence of swelling and ecchymosis. The upward displacement of prostate on digital examination is another indicator of urethral injury. In a suspected child of urethral injury, one should attempt catheterization; otherwise partial disruption may become a complete disruption or may lead to creation of a false passage. Imaging of urethral injury is usually done by retrograde urethrograph. The indicators of urethral injury are filling defect, extravasation of dye, or elongation of urethra [16].

The urethral injuries are classified as (1) contusions, (2) stretch injuries, and (3) disruptions – partial and complete. The injuries can be classified on RGU (retrograde urethrography). Grade I and II injuries are a filling defect seen due to contusion and hematoma or an elongated urethra without any evidence of extravasation of contrast. Grade III injuries are extravasation of same contrast from urethra but maintained bladder continuity. Grade IV injury is extravasation of contrast in urethra with no bladder outline. The posterior urethral injury carries poor prognosis, and its complications include incontinence, retrograde ejaculation, impotence, and urethral strictures. The complications may occur due to injury itself or due to iatrogenic cause following surgical repair [17].

The emergency management of the most of the posterior urethral injuries is conservative. In fact, grade I or II injuries, where the patients are able to evacuate, may not even need catheterization. However only per urethral catheterization is the only treatment for the rest of the grade I and II injury patients. If per urethral catheter is not passable, suprapubic catheter is inserted. For more severe injuries, the best results are achieved in staged procedure; the initial procedure is to divert the urine via suprapubic catheterization followed by definitive repair. The other options are primary surgical repair which involves freshening of the urethral ends and anastomosis of the disrupted urethral ends. The ends can be realigned over a catheter or by endoscopic and radiologic techniques followed by delayed urethroplasty. Primary surgical repair carries high risk of dreaded complications associated with posterior urethral repair like incontinence and impotence besides severe bleeding in acute setting.

To avoid impotency and urinary incontinence, suprapubic cystostomy with delayed urethroplasty is advocated. This carries the risk of urethral stricture until the patient is taken up for definitive repair of the posterior urethra, but this risk is acceptable when compared to other debilitating complications like impotence and incontinence. It also has the advantage of controlled blood loss [18].

Injury to anterior urethra is suspected on retrograde urethrogram if there is depiction of minimal contrast extravasation in anterior urethra with retained ability of the patient to void urine without any difficulty. Almost all patients of grade I or II only require a per urethral catheter drainage only if at all. The patients who are voiding without difficulty do not require even catheter drainage. The grade II and III injuries are managed by per urethral catheter drainage. The grade IV injuries are managed by staged procedure, i.e., placement of a suprapubic catheter followed by delayed urethroplasty.

Urethral injury is rare in girls. The common mechanism of injury is straddle injury, and the most common mode is motor vehicle accidents. The forms of injury encountered in girls are complete avulsion from its attachment to perineal body or disruptions and lacerations at introitus. The proximal disruptions are mostly associated with bladder neck injury and associated pelvic and vaginal injury. Because of short urethral length in females, urethrography is difficult and inconclusive. These patients should be subjected to urethroscopy. Proximal injuries require bladder neck and vaginal repair, while distal injuries can be managed with extended per urethral catheter drainage. The long-term complications seen in girls with urethral injury are urethrovaginal fistula, urethral stenosis, vaginal stenosis, and incontinence [17]. Misdiagnosis or delayed diagnosis is associated with more chances of these complications.

References

1. Brown SL, Elder JS, Spirnak JP. Are pediatric patients more susceptible to major renal injury from blunt trauma? A comparative study. J Urol. 1998;160(1):138–40.
2. Santucci RA, McAninch JW. Diagnosis and management of renal trauma; past, present, and future. J Am Coll Surg. 2000;191(4):443–51.

3. Fraser JD, Aguayo P, Ostlie DJ, St Peter SD. Review of the evidence on the management of blunt renal trauma in pediatric patients. Pediatr Surg Int. 2009;25(2):125–32.
4. Umbreit EC, Routh JC, Husmann DA. Nonoperative management of nonvascular grade IV blunt renal trauma in children: meta-analysis and systematic review. Urology. 2009;74(3):579–82.
5. Tinkoff G, Esposito TJ, Reed J, et al. American Association for the Surgery of Trauma Organ Injury Scale I: spleen, liver, and kidney, validation based on the National Trauma Data Bank. J Am Coll Surg. 2008;207:646–55.
6. Kiankhooy A, Sartorelli KH, Vane DW, Bhave AD. Angiographic embolization is safe and effective therapy for blunt abdominal solid organ injury in children. J Trauma. 2010;68(3):526–31.
7. Fuchs ME, Anderson RE, Myers JB, Wallis MC. The incidence of long-term hypertension in children after high-grade renal trauma. J Pediatr Surg. 2015;50(11):1919–21.
8. Nance ML, Lutz N, Carr MC, et al. Blunt renal injuries in children can be managed nonoperatively: outcome in a consecutive series of patients. J Trauma. 2004;57:474–8.
9. Sims CA, Wiebe DJ, Nance ML. Blunt solid organ injury: do adult and pediatric surgeons treat children differently? J Trauma. 2008;65:698–703.
10. Gaines BA. Intra-abdominal solid organ injury in children: diagnosis and treatment. J Trauma. 2009;67(2 Suppl):S135–9.
11. Dervan LA, King MA, Cuschieri J, Rivara FP, Weiss NS. Pediatric solid organ injury operative interventions and outcomes at Harborview Medical Center, before and after introduction of a solid organ injury pathway for pediatrics. J Trauma Acute Care Surg. 2015;79(2):215–20.
12. Notrica DM. Pediatric blunt abdominal trauma: current management. Curr Opin Crit Care. 2015;21(6):531–7.
13. Puapong D, Brown CV, Katz M, et al. Angiography and the pediatric trauma patient: a 10-year review. J Pediatr Surg. 2006;41:1859–63.
14. Wessells H, Suh D, Porter JR, et al. Renal injury and operative management in the United States: results of a population-based study. J Trauma. 2003;54:423–30.
15. Margenthaler JA, Weber TR, Keller MS. Blunt renal trauma in children: experience with conservative management at a pediatric trauma center. J Trauma. 2002;52:928–32.
16. Wessel LM, Scholz S, Jester I, et al. Management of kidney injuries in children with blunt abdominal trauma. J Pediatr Surg. 2000;35:1326–30.
17. Elshihabi I, Elshihabi S, Arar M. An overview of renal trauma. Curr Opin Pediatr. 1998;10:162–6.
18. Keller MS, Coln CE, Weber TR, et al. Injury grade predicts functional outcome in nonoperatively managed renal injuries in children. Abstract presented at the 34th Annual Meeting of the American Pediatric Surgical Association. May 25–28, 2003.

Blunt Bowel Injuries in Children

12

Rizwan Ahmad Khan

12.1 Introduction

Intestinal injury is less commonly seen than solid organ injury in blunt abdominal trauma. There is 1–15% reported incidence of intestinal injury in children with blunt trauma. Since its incidence is not so common, a high index of suspicion is required for its diagnosis and better prognosis. The jejunum is the most common site of intestinal injury, particularly near the ligament of Treitz followed by the ileum, duodenum, colon, and stomach in that order.

The most common mode of injury leading to intestinal injury is motor vehicle accidents. Others include fall from height, struck by bull horn, bicycle handle bar injury, and seat belt injury. Although the increase use of seat belt has resulted in lowering mortality in children from road traffic accidents, it has led to associated increase in rates of intestinal injuries. These injuries, sometimes known as lap belt complex, result from compression of bowel between the hyperflexed lumbar spine and the belt. The incidence of intestinal injuries in lap belt complex may be as high as 50%. The risk of sustaining this type of injury becomes even higher when the belt is worn in loose manner as it happens in small children with bigger seat belt so that it wraps around only in the lap region.

The children with signs suggestive of lap belt injury, e.g., the transverse abdominal ecchymosis call for careful observation [1, 2].

12.2 Mechanisms

There are three different mechanisms of intestinal injury in blunt trauma. These include (1) shearing force injury to small bowel particularly at the sites of bowel

R. A. Khan
Department of Pediatric Surgery, Jawaharlal Nehru Medical College, AMU,
Aligarh, Uttar Pradesh, India

fixity, i.e., the ligament of Treitz and ileocecal region ileum and also rectosigmoid, (2) compression injury due to compression of bowel and mesentery between the abdominal wall and the vertebrae, and (3) rupture and disruption of bowel due to a sudden increase in intrabowel pressure.

The various types of bowel injuries that can occur are (1) contusion, (2) serosal lacerations, (3) perforation, and (4) mesenteric tear.

12.3   Investigating a Blunt Bowel Injury

The diagnosis of bowel injury in children of blunt abdominal trauma is difficult, and it requires good clinical acumen and high index of suspicion. In polytrauma injuries or head injury with impaired consciousness, the diagnosis is still more difficult. The delay in diagnosis of bowel injury leads to increased morbidity and mortality [3]. Complication rates increase after delayed repair of bowel and include wound infection and dehiscence, sepsis, abscess, collection, etc. This is particularly so if the diagnosis has been delayed for more than 24–48 h. The diagnosis is however difficult due to lack of clear early clinical or imaging features. Computed tomography (CT) which is taken as the gold standard imaging tool for evaluation of these trauma victims has undoubtedly decreased the number of laparotomies but has increased the risk of missing bowel and mesenteric injury. Since unnoticed bowel injury and the resulting sepsis may prove fatal, timely and accurate diagnosis is paramount for better patient outcomes. Clinical examination may be non-revealing in comatose patients or patients with multiple injuries. Head or other severe injuries may also complicate the picture. The presence of abdominal tenderness is not a very specific sign and alone is not predictive of an abdominal injury. A clear history of how the injury was sustained is often very helpful. Correct interpretation of clinical signs and symptoms, appropriately applied imaging modality, and precise clinical acumen are required to prevent the unnecessary delay and management of these injuries.

Serial clinical examination is extremely helpful in the diagnosis of small bowel injury. This must be undertaken in all blunt abdominal injuries especially in patients with other associated solid organ injuries, head injury, and hemodynamic instability. A thorough inspection for signs of "seat belt sign" must be made. The most frequent clinical signs associated with bowel injury are abdominal pain as the presenting symptom and abdominal tenderness as the clinical sign. The other indicators of gastrointestinal injury are (1) fever, (2) hematemesis or blood-stained nasogastric aspirates, (3) increasing pulse rate, (4) increasing abdominal distention and tenderness, and (5) development of paralytic ileus [4].

The presence of pancreatic injury is associated with a significantly higher rate of bowel injury.

A plain abdominal X-ray in erect position that shows free gas remains the most consistent indicator of bowel injury. On left lateral decubitus position, there will be evidence of free air trapped between the liver and right hemidiaphragm. The diagnostic value of plain radiograph has been variously reported to vary from 40% to 70%, and also it is rapid and affordable investigation. However, the absence of pneumoperitoneum is not a marker of absent bowel injury.

On ultrasonography, thickening of the bowel wall and heterogenous echogenic thickened bowel wall due to contusion or ineffective peristalsis or ileus may be seen. But this requires extensive knowledge and skill of a highly competent and experienced ultrasonologist particularly because of poor visualization due to bowel gas in ileus [2].

In past, diagnostic peritoneal lavage (DPL) used to be the tool of choice for surgeons for evaluating blunt abdominal injury. It basically evaluated the presence of hemoperitoneum. But with the advent of CT imaging, its use has become obsolete. The major advantages of CT include noninvasiveness, cross-sectional imaging, good visibility of both intraperitoneal and retroperitoneal organs, and short time required for investigation. The CT findings which suggest blunt bowel injury are free fluid, bowel wall thickening or enhancement, extraluminal air, mesenteric stranding, or extravasation of contrast. Presence of free peritoneal fluid with no visible solid organ injury is an important indicator of bowel and mesenteric injury [4].

The use of use of pediatric laparoscopy is nowadays coming up as a minimally invasive technique [5]. Diagnostic laparoscopy may give significant lead while evaluating children with suspicious gastrointestinal perforation following abdominal trauma. As frequency of laparoscopy and thereby expertise in pediatric laparoscopy increase, negative laparotomies can be decreased [6]. Most solid organ injuries are treated conservatively in the pediatric population. In a child with free peritoneal fluid without any other evidence of solid organ injury, the cause of free fluid can be cleared with laparoscopy. Laparoscopy can be both diagnostic and therapeutic [7, 8].

Shock or hemodynamic instability following blunt abdominal trauma may influence the approach and outcome in the early post injury period. In these patients damage control laparotomy is done where the goal is resuscitation, control of hemorrhage, reversal of coagulopathy, and acidosis; contamination from intestinal perforation is limited to stapling of perforations with definitive repair planned after 48–72 h when the patient is stabilized.

12.4 Stomach

Gastric injury in children may occur following handle bar injury or motor vehicle accident. The usual injury is perforation on anterior wall. The presence of rupture requires considerable pressure as occurs in sudden increases in intragastric pressure with compression of the abdomen which leads to rupture over anterior surface or greater curvature of the stomach. When rupture is present, then a search for other visceral injuries should also be made. Thus gastric injuries require thorough exploration. The gastroesophageal junction should be explored and that may necessitate mobilizing the lateral part of the left lobe of the liver. The injury to the gastroesophageal region should raise suspicion of injury to the closely related aorta or celiac trunk. The lesser sac should be explored to inspect the posterior wall of stomach and to rule out pancreatic injury. Another important structure closely related to the stomach that requires inspection is the diaphragm. The edges of the gastric injury should be debrided and repair performed with a simple two layers. If there is injury to the vagus nerve or extensive damage to the pylorus, pyloroplasty may be required. A severe avulsion injury at gastroduodenal region may require antrectomy. Gastric resection is rare required especially in blunt injury. The postoperative care necessitates a nasogastric tube drainage for several days [9].

12.5 Duodenum

Duodenal injury following blunt trauma may result due to direct blunt force or due to compression against the vertebral column. Subserosal hemorrhage from blunt injury produces a duodenal hematoma that may lead to partial or complete obstruction. It may require gastric decompression and total parenteral nutrition and typically resolves spontaneously over 1–3 weeks. The management of duodenal perforation is governed by the extent of injury and presence of associated pancreatic injury. A Kocher maneuver should be performed in order to allow for complete inspection of both the duodenum and head of the pancreas. Most of the duodenal perforations are treatable by primary repair. If the size is large, then proximal and distal drainage and distal feeding jejunostomy may be required. Pyloric exclusion can be useful in extensive pancreaticoduodenal injuries. Complete resection or diverticulization is rarely necessary [9, 10].

12.6 Mesentery

The mesenteric injuries are important as they may cause segmental areas of ischemia. More importantly they are the most common cause of delayed presentation of intestinal injury. Mesenteric involvement must be searched for hematomas, linear or transverse lacerations, and hernias (Fig. 12.1). The bleeding should be controlled, the defects should be repaired, and the viability of the associated bowel should be checked before closure [11].

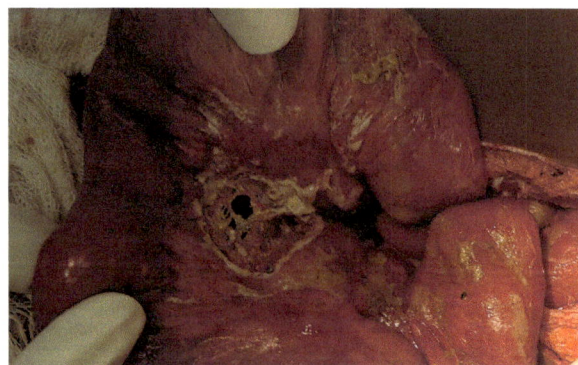

Fig. 12.1 Mesentric injury showing transverse laceration

12.7   Small Bowel

Ileal and jejunal injuries can occur anywhere along their length; however there is great propensity of involvement at points of relative fixity, i.e., ligament of Treitz and ileocecal junction. The management of these small bowel injuries in children is similar to adults. Thorough inspection of whole small and large bowel and mesentery should be done. The majority of bowel injuries occur on the antimesenteric border (Fig. 12.2). Full-thickness injuries but involving less than half of the circumference of the bowel should be debrided and repaired in a transverse manner in two layers. If the injury involves more than 50% the circumference, it requires resection and anastomosis. The management of colonic injuries (Fig. 12.3) is governed by the

Fig. 12.2 Blunt injury to jejunum

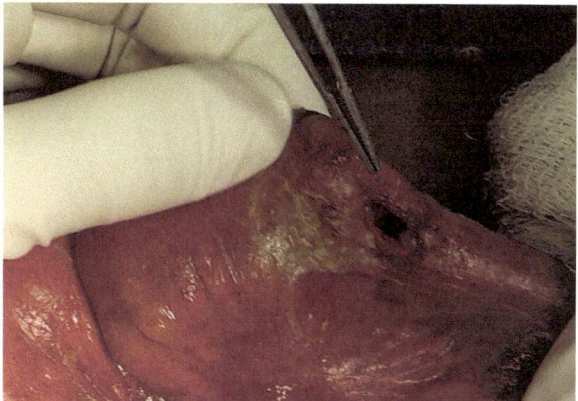

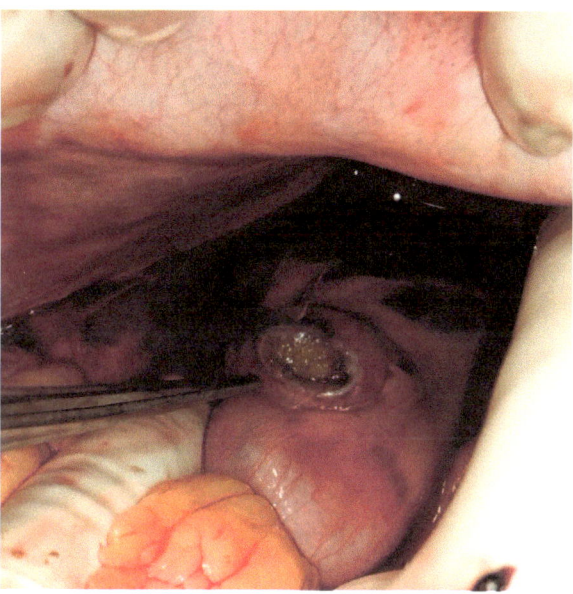

Fig. 12.3 Blunt injury to colon

presence of abdominal contamination and delay in taking up the case. Nowadays the trend is toward primary repair as many randomized studies suggest that primary repair is not only equal but preferable to colostomy. In cases where there is early (6 h) and minimal contamination, primary repair is preferable to diversion. The presence of multiple injuries or comorbid conditions correlates with a higher failure rate in primary repair. In distal colonic injuries or rectal injuries with peritoneal involvement, colostomy may be appropriate [12].

In children with anorectal injury, primary repair with colostomy is the preferred approach.

A late sequel of blunt intestinal injury is intestinal stricture. The most frequent mechanism is localized area of crush injury or contusion to the bowel wall, which causes ischemic injury and ensuing fibrosis. Stricture may also occur at primary repair or anastomosis site. Adhesive bowel obstruction is another important presentation in these children. These patients present with nausea and bilious emesis, 1–6 weeks after the primary intervention. The most common mode of management is conservative [13].

References

1. Nance ML, Keller MS, Stafford PW. Predicting hollow visceral injury in the pediatric blunt trauma patient with solid visceral injury. J Pediatr Surg. 2000;35:1300–3.
2. Holland AJ, Cass DT, Glasson MJ, et al. Small bowel injuries in children. J Paediatr Child Health. 2000;36:265–9.
3. Paris C, Brindamour M, Ouimet A, St-Vil D. Predictive indicators for bowel injury in pediatric patients who present with a positive seat belt sign after motor vehicle collision. J Pediatr Surg. 2010;45:921–4.
4. Hom J. The risk of intra-abdominal injuries in pediatric patients with stable blunt abdominal trauma and negative abdominal computed tomography. Acad Emerg Med. 2010;17:469–75.
5. Bixby SD, Callahan MJ, Taylor GA. Imaging in pediatric blunt abdominal trauma. Semin Roentgenol. 2008;43:72–82.
6. VanderKolk WE, Garcia VF. The use of laparoscopy in the management of seat belt trauma in children. J Laparoendosc Surg. 1996;6:S45–9.
7. McKinley AJ, Mahomed AA. Laparoscopy in a case of pediatric blunt abdominal trauma. Surg Endosc. 2002;16:358.
8. Gandhi RR, Stringel G. Laparoscopy in pediatric abdominal trauma. JSLS. 1997;1:349–51.
9. Ulman I, Avanoglu A, Ozcan C, et al. Gastrointestinal perforations in children: a continuing challenge to nonoperative treatment of blunt abdominal trauma. J Trauma. 1996;41:110–3.
10. Ozturk H, Onen A, Otcu S, et al. Diagnostic delay increases morbidity in children with gastrointestinal perforation from blunt abdominal trauma. Surg Today. 2003;33:178–82.
11. Sarihan H, Abes M. Non-operative management of intraabdominal bleeding due to blunt trauma in children: the risk of associated intestinal injuries. Pediatr Surg Int. 1998;13:108–11.
12. Schimpl G, Schmidt B, Sauer H. Isolated bowel injury in blunt abdominal trauma in childhood. Eur J Pediatr Surg. 1992;2:341–4.
13. Thompson SR, Holland AJA. Perforating small bowel injuries in children: influence of time to operative operation on outcome. Injury. 2005;36:1029–33.

13

Manal Mohd Khan

13.1 Traumatic Abdominal Wall Defects and Reconstruction in Paediatric Patients

Abdominal injuries following trauma are the third most common (after head injury and extremity). In paediatric population, other causes of acquired abdominal wall defects are previous surgery, infection and tumour resection. We will discuss post-traumatic abdominal wall injuries including degloving injuries and their management. The aims of reconstruction in abdominal wall injuries are to shielding of the abdominal viscera and restoration of functional capacity of the abdominal wall [1, 2]. The reconstruction of complex defects can be quite demanding and requires close collaboration between plastic and paediatric surgeons.

13.2 Surgical Anatomy

When planning abdominal wall reconstruction, an overlook at the surgical perspective of anatomy of the abdominal wall is important.

13.2.1 Skin and Subcutaneous Tissue

The epidermis is the outermost layer, which provides the major barrier and is supported and nourished by the underlying dermis which also contains nerves, vessels and appendages: sweat glands, hair follicles and sebaceous glands. Subcutaneous fat forms the third and deepest layer of the skin. The underlying subcutaneous tissue has two layers; superficial and deep layers. In between these two layers there is

M. M. Khan
Department of Plastic Surgery, AIIMS, Bhopal, Madhya Pradesh, India

© Springer Nature Singapore Pte Ltd. 2018
R. Ahmad Khan, S. Wahab (eds.), *Blunt Abdominal Trauma in Children*,
https://doi.org/10.1007/978-981-13-0692-1_13

Scarpa's fascia. The superficial subcutaneous layer spans the whole abdominal wall, while the deep subcutaneous layer covers only the lower abdomen, inferior to the umbilicus level [3]. For an optimal aesthetic outcome, the continuity amongst the contents of the subcutaneous tissues has to be maintained [4, 5].

13.2.2 Musculofascial Layers

A familiarity and comprehensive knowledge of the different strata of the abdominal wall and its overlapping layers and their realignments are very important in planning reconstruction of the wall. The fascial layers fuse and form three distinct anatomic lines on the abdominal wall. The linea alba is a white dense line in the midline of abdomen while there are two semilunar lines which run along the lateral border of rectus abdominis. The deep fascia of the abdomen is formed by the fusion of the aponeuroses of the oblique muscles of the abdominal wall: internal and external oblique. The semilunar line formed by the fusion of transversus abdominis at the lateral margin of the rectus muscle. The anterior fascial layer is formed by the fusion of the aponeuroses of the oblique muscles of the abdominal wall above the arcuate line. The aponeurosis of the internal oblique divides and unites with the transverses abdominis on the posterior aspect of the rectus abdominis muscle to form the posterior layer. This posterior fascial layer outlines the abdomen and separates abdominal wall from the peritoneum. Inferior to the arcuate line, the aponeuroses of the three flat muscles of the abdomen are fused together and strengthen the anterior layer of the rectus sheath [6, 7]. The abdominal wall musculature is divided into anterior, anterolateral and posterior layers. The anterior layer is formed by the rectus abdominis and pyramidalis muscles; the anterolateral layer is formed by the external oblique, internal oblique and transversus abdominis muscles; and posterior layer is composed of the quadratus lumborum muscle [4, 6, 7].

13.2.3 Vascular Supply

The abdominal wall is mainly supplied by two sources; cutaneous vessels and musculocutaneous vessels [8]. Huger has given a classification of the vascular supply of abdominal wall by dividing it into simple zones. He originally classified it for use excision of abdominal fat (abdominal lipectomy) in morbidly obese patients [9]. However this classification has become useful for planning reconstruction algorithms of the abdominal wall.

Zone I is the midabdomen region around the umbilicus. The chief vascular supply of this region is from the deep epigastric arcade which is formed by the superior and inferior epigastric arteries. Superficial epigastric artery originates from the internal thoracic artery and moves down along the posterior rectus sheath, while the deep inferior epigastric artery after branching off the external iliac artery moves up along the posterior rectus sheath. Both the vessels during their course supply the rectus abdominis and the associated skin.

Zone II is the region of lower abdomen and is chiefly supplied by the blood vessels which arise from the epigastric arcade and the external iliac artery. The femoral artery gives off the superficial epigastric and superficial external pudendal arteries which then travel superficial to the fascia and supplying the above skin. The muscles of the Zone II receive their blood supply through the inferior epigastric artery which runs on the posterior rectus sheath supplying the branches to the adjoining muscles. However the muscles around the anterior iliac spine receive their blood supply from the deep circumflex iliac artery.

Zone III is the region of the flanks and lateral abdomen. The intercostal, subcostal and lumbar arteries provide the chief arterial supply to the Zone III. These vessels are the branches of the aorta. They course along the lateral abdominal wall circumferentially on the transversus abdominis and through the oblique muscles and supply the overlying skin.

The *lymphatics* of the abdominal wall very much like the arterial supply have the similar distribution but have many overlaps in their distribution. In Zone II (i.e. inferior to the umbilicus), the lymphatics drain into the inguinal nodes. The deeper areas are drained into the external iliac nodes. Zone III is drained into the lateral lumbar nodes and superficial inguinal nodes. Zone I is drained into external iliac nodes, lateral lumbar nodes and superficial inguinal nodes [9, 10].

13.2.4 Innervation

The nerve roots T7–L4 supply the motor and sensory innervation to the abdomen through the following nerves: subcostal, intercostal, ilioinguinal nerves and iliohypogastric nerves. The course of these nerves is circumferential along the lateral abdominal wall and finally ending in the midline of anterior abdomen. The outer layer formed by the external oblique is supplied by the intercostal, subcostal and iliohypogastric nerves. The middle and the inner muscles, i.e. the internal oblique and transversus abdominis muscles, receive their nerve supply via the intercostal, subcostal, iliohypogastric and ilioinguinal nerves. The rectus abdominis muscle receives its innervation through five lower intercostal nerves and the subcostal nerve. The iliohypogastric nerve supplies sensory signals to the region of pubis with some intersection from the femoral cutaneous nerve. During reconstruction these nerves should be preserved both for maintaining sensory function as well as the motor function [4, 9].

13.3 Mechanism of Injury

The most common mechanism injuring the abdominal wall is blunt trauma which occurs in 90% of the patients. These include motor vehicle accidents, fall from height and bicycle-related injuries. In about 10% of cases, penetrating injuries like gunshot, sharps and impalement of sharp objects are the cause. In children with blunt injury, there are more chances of associated intra-abdominal injury as compared to penetrating [12].

Degloving soft-tissue injuries (DSTIs) are defined as avulsion or detachment of the skin and the associated subcutaneous tissue from the musculofascial layer lying underneath. This injury usually occurs as result of sudden application of shearing force over the abdominal wall. It can involve any part of the body, and the main sites are the abdomen, lower limbs, face and scalp. These may be associated with variable amount of skin and subcutaneous tissue loss [13, 14]. DSTIs are of two types: open or closed. The open DSTIs are characterized by the severing of the skin off the body, and some portion with or without subcutaneous tissue may remain attached to the body. Closed DSTI is rare, and it occurs as a consequence of direct force with tangential impact leading to separation of skin and subcutaneous tissue from the adjoining muscles, but the integrity of the skin is maintained and creates a cavity underneath. This is also known as Morel-Lavallée lesion and because of the cavity it accumulates hematoma, lymph, and viable and necrotic liquefied tissue [13–15].

Objectives of abdominal reconstruction:

1. To re-establish the function and integrity of the musculofascial abdominal planes
2. To prevent evisceration of intrabdominal viscera
3. To restore dynamic support of abdominal muscles [4, 11]

13.3.1 Diagnosis

Diagnosis of abdominal wall injuries is a challenging task. Clinical assessment of abdominal wall is the first step, but may not predict exact extent of the injury. Intravenous dye like fluorescein may be used to estimate the line of demarcation between healthy and dead tissue. Open degloving soft-tissue injuries (DSTIs) are usually self-descriptive of the nature and extent of injury. These are associated with overlying ecchymosis, abrasion or other wounds in and around the main wound [13]. If complete avulsion is present, then colour, temperature, capillary refill time and bleeding from the margins are the indicators of the viability of the flap. Morel-Lavallée lesion diagnosis is frequently diagnosed late because of unpredictable clinical presentation, and the superficial skin presentation may mask the real lesion. High-resolution ultrasonography and computed tomography (CT) have been used to diagnose the lesion, but MRI is considered as the radiological investigation of choice for proper assessment of wall lesions and Morel-Lavallée lesions [16, 17].

13.4 Management

The acute management of the severely injured child is discussed in Chaps. 5 and 6. The abdominal wall lesions are usually detected in *secondary survey* which is a head-to-toe examination or may be later in *tertiary survey* where the rest of the missed or hidden injuries are identified.

The primary management for airway and haemodynamic stability should be performed as per the protocol. Survey evaluation for the extent of the abdominal injuries should be carried out as for the other injuries in all the patients.

The common aim of all surgical approaches is to re-establish abdominal wall cover.

13.4.1 Preparation of Wound Bed

Thorough examination of the injured area is carried out at initial evaluation. The avulsion injury of abdominal wall may initially appear salvageable, but it may not be the case as the true extent of the injury may be reflected in early stage of the injury. The abdominal skin receives its blood supply from a rich plexus of small vessels which is supplied by the perforators arising from the underlying musculofascial plane. Consequently, the degloving injuries lead to tearing off of these perforators and thereby hampering the blood supply of the degloved abdominal wall which after sometime of injury may become nonviable [19]. The accompanying venous vessels are also affected leading to incomplete venous drainage and resultant subsequent venous congestion. The interrupted arterial supply together with increased venous congestion pressure across the abdominal wall skin plexuses ultimately leads to flap necrosis [19]. Therefore, if primary closure of such wounds is tried, these flaps frequently have high incidence of necrosis which may progress to severe wound sepsis [20]. Delineation of nonviable areas (mostly the distal most tips) of the flap becomes generally obvious after 24 h. The ultimate extent of necrosis of the flap is generally confirmed by fifth or seventh day following the injury. Before the reconstruction, the wound bed must be clean so that there are negligible exudates and healthy margins of the degloved skin flaps/abdominal wall defects [21].

For the better soft-tissue management, the principles are to decrease the tissue loss and reduce the wound contamination. Serial excision (debridement) of devitalized tissue is performed till the wound bed is healthy and ready for reconstruction [21].

13.4.2 Reconstruction: Immediate Versus Delayed

The decision to reconstruct immediately or on delayed basis depends on the clinical presentation and condition of patient. It is preferable to do immediate reconstruction as it is cost effective as well as time saving. This is feasible in clinically stable patients with adequate wound bed and availability of reconstructive options. Delayed reconstruction is preferred if the patient is clinically unstable, having inadequate or uncertain reconstructive options, the wound bed is not healthy, or additional operative procedures are planned. The results may be better with a staged procedure which allows preservation of more tissue [2, 18, 21] (Tables 13.1 and 13.2).

Table 13.1 Repair of partial abdominal wall defects

	Partial defects			
	Myofascial defect			
	Autologous reconstruction			Non-autologous reconstruction
Skin defect	Upper 1/3	Middle 1/3	Lower 1/3	
Primary closure (<5 cm) Skin grafts Local/random flaps Fasciocutaneous flaps Vacuum assisted closure (VAC/NPWT) Tissue expansion	(a) *Small (central <10 cm lateral <5 cm)* primary closure comp septn local flaps (sup rect. abd, Ext. Oblique) (b) *Large (central >10 cm lateral >5 cm)* distant flaps (ext. TFL, RF, LD) Tissue expansion FTT	(a) *Small (central <6 cm lateral <3 cm)* primary closure comp septn local flaps (sup rect. abd, Ext. Oblique) (b) *Large (central >6 cm lateral >3 cm)* distant flaps (TFL, RF) Tissue expansion FTT	(a) *Small (central <20 cm lateral <10 cm)* primary closure comp septn local flaps (Inf. rect. abd, Int. Oblique) (b) *Large (central >20 cm lateral >10 cm)* distant flaps (TFL, RF, vastus lateralis, gracilis) Tissue expansion FTT	Prosthetic reconstruction

TFL tensor fasciae latae, *RF* rectus femoris, *LD* lattissimus dorsi, *FTT* free tissue transfer

Table 13.2 Repair of complete abdominal wall defects

	Complete defects			
	Inadequate skin			
Adequate skin (<15 cm)	Immediate reconstruction			Delayed reconstruction
	Upper 1/3	Middle 1/3	Lower 1/3	
Musculofascial defect (manage as partial defect, see Table 13.1)	Local flaps/skin graft (Sup rect. abd, Ext. Olique) Distant flaps (Extended LD, Extended TFL) Prosthesis/Flap Tissue expansion Free tissue transfer	Local flaps/skin graft (Sup rect. abd, Ext. Olique) Distant flaps (TFL, RF) Prosthesis/Flap Tissue expansion Free tissue transfer	Local flaps/skin graft (Inf. rect. abd, Int. Olique) Distant flaps (TFL, RF, Vastus Lateralis, Gracilis) Prosthesis/Flap Tissue expansion Free tissue transfer	Prosthetic reconstruction Delayed skin graft

TFL tensor fasciae latae, *RF* rectus femoris, *LD* lattissimus dorsi

References

1. Gaines BA, Ford HR. Abdominal and pelvic trauma in children. Crit Care Med. 2002;30:416–23.
2. Rohrich RJ, Lowe JB, Hackney FL, Bowman JL, Hobar PC. An algorithm for abdominal wall reconstruction. Plast Reconstr Surg. 2000;105:202–16.
3. Markman B. Anatomy and physiology of adipose tissue. Clin Plast Surg. 1989;16:235.
4. Core GB, Grotting JC. Reoperative surgery of the abdominal wall. In: Grotting JC, editor. Aesthetic and reconstructive plastic surgery, vol. 2. St. Louis: Quality Medical Publishing, Inc.; 1995. p. 1327–75.
5. Lockwood TE. Superficial fascial system (SFS) of the trunk and extremities: a new concept. Plast Reconstr Surg. 1991;87:1009.
6. Netter FH. Atlas of human anatomy. Summit, NJ: Ciba-Geigy; 1989.
7. Chung KW. Gross anatomy. Baltimore: Williams and Wilkins; 1988. p. 159–204.
8. Nahai F, Brown RG, Vasconez LO. Blood supply to the abdominal wall as related to planning abdominal incisions. Am Surg. 1976;42:691.
9. Huger WE Jr. The anatomic rationale for abdominal lipectomy. Am Surg. 1979;45:612.
10. Burns AJ. Trunk reconstruction (overview). Sel Read Plast Surg. 1995;7:1.
11. DiBello JN Jr, Moore JH. Sliding myofascial flap of the rectus abdominis muscles for closure of recurrent ventral hernias. Plast Reconstr Surg. 1996;98:464.
12. Sinha CK, Lander A. Trauma in children: abdomen and thorax. Surgery (Oxford). 2013;31(3):123–9.
13. Morris M, Schreiber MA, Ham B. Novel management of closed degloving injuries. J Trauma. 2009;67:E121–3.
14. Mello DF, Assef JC, Soldá SC, Helene A Jr. Degloving injuries of trunk and limbs: comparison of outcomes of early versus delayed assessment by the plastic surgery team. Rev Col Bras Cir. 2015;42:143–8. https://doi.org/10.1590/0100-69912015003003.
15. Luta V, Enache A, Costea C. Posttraumatic Morel-Lavallée seroma – clinic and forensic implications. Rom J Leg Med. 2010;18(1):31–6.
16. Arnez ZM, Khan U, Tyler MP. Classification of soft-tissue degloving in limb trauma. J Plast Reconstr Aesthet Surg. 2010;63(11):1865–9.
17. Rha EY, Kim DH, Kwon H, Jung SN. Morel-lavallee lesion in children. World J Emerg Surg. 2013;8:60. http://www.wjes.org/content/8/1/60
18. Gottlieb JR, Engrav LH, Walkinshaw MD, Eddy AC, Herman CM. Upper abdominal wall defects: immediate or staged reconstruction? Plast Reconstr Surg. 1990;86:281.
19. De Korte N, Dwars BJ, van der Werff JF. Degloving injury of an extremity. Is primary closure obsolete? J Trauma. 2009;67:60–1.
20. Kudsk KA, Sheldon GF, Walton RL. Degloving injuries of the extremities and torso. J Trauma. 1981;21:835–9.
21. Lau J, Lim X, Chen OW, Lin YY, Lim J, et al. A case report of traumatic perineal degloving injury. Surgery Curr Res. 2017;7:284. https://doi.org/10.4172/2161-1076.1000284.

Rizwan Ahmad Khan and Shagufta Wahab

14.1 Perineal Injuries

Injuries to the anorectum, external genitalia, and urethra are rare in children but when present are associated with significant morbidity. Most of the perineal injuries in children are due to penetrating trauma. The perineal injuries are sustained either from accident or sexual abuse. Injuries sustained by sexual abuse generally involve the rectum or vagina with evidences of forceful penetrations. However accidental penetrating injuries to the perineum involve all the structures without any predilection for orifice involvement [1]. The blunt injuries to the perineum are usually sustained by straddle injuries. This may lead to bruising and contusion in and around perineal structures.

The assessment of these injuries requires thorough examination under anesthesia. It includes cystoscopy, genitoscopy, proctoscopy, and sigmoidoscopy. The nature, extent of injury, and any laceration and its depth should be confirmed. If required it should be supplemented with retrograde urethrogram or lower gastrointestinal contrast study. A careful abdominal examination should also be done to rule out associated intra-abdominal injuries.

14.1.1 Boys

Penile injuries are rare either following blunt or penetrating trauma in children. The clinical findings of excessive bleeding, an increasing hematoma, or a palpable

R. A. Khan (✉)
Department of Pediatric Surgery, Jawaharlal Nehru Medical College, AMU, Aligarh, Uttar Pradesh, India

S. Wahab
Department of Radiodiagnosis, Jawaharlal Nehru Medical College, AMU, Aligarh, Uttar Pradesh, India

© Springer Nature Singapore Pte Ltd. 2018
R. Ahmad Khan, S. Wahab (eds.), *Blunt Abdominal Trauma in Children*,
https://doi.org/10.1007/978-981-13-0692-1_14

121

corporal defect indicate cavernosal injuries. Large cavernosal injuries require primary repair. Penile injuries following zipper entrapment can be mostly managed with local anesthetic and only sometimes may need a general anesthetic for the release of the penis [2]. Injury from hair tourniquets may lead to penile strangulation and may result in necrosis of the prepucial skin, glans, distal penile skin, cavernosum, or urethra. These injuries are common sources of constriction and may be quite difficult to remove. Most of these injuries require planned approach as injuries are usually chronic in nature.

Since the testicles are mobile organ, blunt injury is rare. Direct blows are the most common mode of blunt injuries with almost 50% of direct blows lead to testicular rupture. Clinically it is often difficult to differentiate between the testicular rupture and simple testicular contusion owing to and associated with reactive hydrocele/hematoceles [1, 2].

Ultrasound is the initial diagnostic modality for assessment of testicular injuries. However, only a classic case of testicular rupture, i.e., a tunica albuginea rupture with extrusion of seminiferous tubule, can be diagnosed with ultrasound. Some authors cite the risk of understaging and therefore do not recommend it (specificity 78%, sensitivity 28%). The presence of hematocele on ultrasound is only suggestive of and not pathognomonic of testicular rupture. Surgical exploration of the testis with evacuation of "large" hematomas in children and adults is recommended as this hastens the recovery. The treatment of blunt testicular and scrotal injuries is controversial. Most of the surgeons prefer conservative approach, while operative intervention involves exploration, debridement, and repair of these ruptures. Those who are the proponents of operative approach argue that conservative management may lead to superimposed infection, atrophy, and increases the risk of orchiectomy on subsequent exploration.

14.1.2 Girls

The blunt perineal and genital injuries in girls occur usually after a straddle injury, e.g., falling with open legs on chair, the seat of bicycle, or parapet wall. These injuries present as contusion, hematoma, or laceration. Other forms of blunt injury to perineum occur after being hit by a stick or ball during a game. Children under the age of 10 are more prone to laceration injuries following falls. Girls are especially prone to injuries following sexual assault. All the perineal structures (vagina, anus, and rectum) are susceptible to injury following sexual assault. The presenting symptoms are pain and bleeding following the injury. The children with genital injuries are anxious, uncomfortable, agitated, and embarrassed making any attempt at examination futile. Therefore it is of utmost importance that all the children with genital injuries must be examined thoroughly under general anesthesia. The treatment of female genital trauma depends on the type and extent of injury. Absorbable sutures are advised to avoid the need for removal [3].

The treatment of perineal injuries involves careful exploration and extirpation of any necrosed tissue. This is followed by anatomical reconstruction which should be done with or without diversion depending upon the injury. Lacerations are primarily repaired after proper hemostasis. The urethral repair should be performed with perurethral catheter or suprapubic cystostomy. The rectal tears are repaired, and complex injuries (involving sphincter) are diverted with sigmoid colostomy. Broad-spectrum antibiotics and tetanus prophylaxis are a must in managing these wounds. The sphincteric function should be assessed after complete wound healing and cor-roborated with detailed radiological confirmation, e.g., intravenous urography, mic-turating cystourethrogram, and distal colography. Any further reconstruction or continuity restoration surgery should be taken after complete wound healing is evi-denced by radiological investigation [4].

14.2   Diaphragmatic Injury

Traumatic diaphragmatic injury is infrequent in children. The usual blunt injury mechanism responsible for diaphragmatic injury is a massive compressive force to the abdominal wall leading to rushing of abdominal contents upward rupturing the diaphragm. The left-sided injuries are more common. However, a series from Toronto had reported that 13 of 15 of their patients had rupture of the diaphragm following blunt trauma; and the right and left diaphragms were equally involved. The patients often have concurrent seatbelt signs and Chance fractures. The diagno-sis of diaphragmatic injury is frequently overlooked. A high index of suspicion for injury to the diaphragm is required in suitable clinical setting, for instance, lateral vehicular accidents more so in left-sided crashes and direct frontal collisions. The diagnosis can be made on dedicated clinical examination which can be confirmed by using chest X-ray. There are two typical signs of diaphragmatic injury on chest radiography. First is the detection of intrathoracic location of a hollow viscus as a mass occupying, mostly on the left side which may or may be associated with a col-lar sign (i.e., conical waist of the displaced bowel due to its compression as it wrings through the diaphragmatic rent). Second is the presence of a nasogastric tube seen on chest X-ray above the left hemidiaphragm. This conventional chest X-ray finding can be seen in almost 60–90% patients presenting with suspected acute traumatic diaphragmatic ruptures. However, these findings are not very specific and cannot be differentiated from hemothorax, atelectasis, etc. Therefore sometimes fluoroscopy, CT scan or mechanical MR imaging may be required. Thin-cut CT scan chest with multiplanar reconstruction improves the detection of diaphragmatic injuries. It clearly demonstrates the intra-abdominal contents adjacent to the posterior thoracic wall and the "collar" sign. The other indications of diaphragmatic injury are "dis-continuous" and thickened diaphragm. Since the force required to cause such an injury is usually massive, other associated injuries should also be suspected. The most commonly injured organs are the liver (laceration), spleen (laceration), bowel (perforation), and pelvis and bone. Primary repair with nonabsorbable suture is usu-ally possible in most of the cases. If enough diaphragmatic tissue is lost after excis-ing the devitalized tissue, then adequate size mesh should be utilized to close the defect [5].

Since diaphragmatic injuries are quite rare, a high index of suspicion is required and calls for observation and palpation of both diaphragms when operating on children with other intra-abdominal injuries particularly upper abdominal injuries.

14.3   Blunt Injuries to Abdominal Vessels

Traumatic disruption of abdominal vessels is rare in blunt abdominal trauma afflicting children, but when present, they can be extremely lethal. The frequency of injury to the major vessels of the abdomen is the aorta, superior mesenteric artery (SMA), iliac arteries, inferior vena cava (IVC), portal vein (PV), and iliac veins in that order. Clinical picture is defined on the resultant effect of the vascular injury, i.e., it has resulted in retroperitoneal hematoma or free intraperitoneal hemorrhage. Rapidly falling blood pressure should arouse the suspicion of large vessel injury, and immediate intravenous access with the largest possible size of venous cannula should be established, appropriate resuscitation with warmed 1:1:1 fluid should be started, and simultaneous preparation for immediate surgical exploration must be planned. The retroperitoneum is separated into three zones according to the location of the major vessels. Zone I extends in the midline of the abdomen and further divided into the supramesocolic and inframesocolic regions. Zone I contains the aorta, IVC, celiac, and superior and inferior mesenteric arteries. Zone II is the area of the bilateral paracolic gutters, i.e., along the ascending and descending colon. Zone II contains the renal vessels and kidneys. The region under the sacral promontory is designated as Zone III, and it contains the iliac arteries and veins [6].

14.3.1 Zone I Retroperitoneal Injuries

14.3.1.1   Aortic Injuries

Several series have reported a mortality rate ranging from 50% to 78% in aortic injuries. In Zone I, injuries to aorta are divided into diaphragmatic, suprarenal, and infrarenal injuries. Injuries to the diaphragmatic aorta presents mostly as contained hematoma rather than free rupture because of the dense connective tissue surrounding this segment of the aorta. Its exposure can be attained via laparotomy and opening into the lesser sac and left anterolateral thoracotomy.

Injuries to the suprarenal abdominal aorta are associated with worse outcomes compared to infrarenal aortic injuries. Proximal control by manual compression or aortic compression device or thoracotomy is the most important before proceeding ahead. For small rent, primary closure, and wider injuries, polytetrafluoroethylene (PTFE), Dacron, or an autologous vein should be used.

Similarly for injuries in the infrarenal abdominal aorta, proximal control can be achieved by applying the aortic clamp just inferior to the origin of the left renal vein or at the diaphragmatic hiatus as previously described before proceeding with repair [6, 7].

14.3.1.2   Inferior Vena Caval (IVC) Injuries

IVC injuries also carry a high morbidity and mortality (36–75%). The classification of the injuries of IVC is based on the site of injury. These are infrarenal, suprarenal, or retrohepatic/suprahepatic. The infrarenal IVC injuries are the easiest to manage. The injuries involving suprarenal IVC require more thorough exposure maneuvers. While repairing these injuries, it should be kept in mind that defects <50% of circumference can be repaired primarily in a transverse fashion, while those which are >50% of the circumference require grafting. Surgical exposure and repair of retrohepatic and suprahepatic IVC injuries are the most challenging and require expertise. Depending upon the injury, this may entail atriocaval shunt or total hepatic isolation (Heaney maneuver) both of which carry a significant mortality [7, 8].

14.3.1.3   Celiac Artery/Superior Mesenteric Artery/Inferior Mesenteric Artery (IMA)

After proper exposure, small injuries can be repaired primarily, while in bigger injuries, the vessel can be ligated safely together with cholecystectomy.

Depending upon the injury site, the injuries of SMA are divided into four zones (Table 14.1) (Fullen classification).

The risk of ischemia is maximal in Zone I SMA injuries, and the risk decreases as we go further down the zones. In a stable patient with SMA injuries, primary repair should be done whenever achievable. Otherwise the options are vein patch angioplasty, interposition graft, and reimplantation. In an unstable patient, if easily possible, the primary repair should be performed, but if not, then the injury can be ligated or shunted.

Inferior mesenteric artery is rarely injured in blunt abdominal injuries. Injuries to IMA can be repaired primarily or ligated with risk of colorectal ischemia.

14.3.1.4   SMV/Portal Vein

Injuries to the portal vein and superior mesenteric veins (SMV) occur rarely and generally due to penetrating trauma. For access Pringle maneuver and Kocher maneuver are widely used. If not repairable then PV should be ligated maintaining the hepatic artery patency. Since ligation of PV carries the risk of splanchnic congestion, consideration should be given to temporary abdominal closure and second-look surgery [9, 10].

Table 14.1 Fullen classification of SMA injuries

Zone	Site of injury to SMA
I	Trunk proximal to first branch
II	Trunk between inferior pancreaticoduodenal and middle colic
III	Trunk distal to middle colic
IV	Segmental branches (jejunal, ileal, colic)

14.3.2 Zone II Retroperitoneal Injuries

Only expanding and/or pulsatile hematomas in Zone II following blunt trauma require exploration. After rotation of viscera, the kidney and hilum are accessed by opening the Gerota's on the lateral aspect. The hilum then is controlled with manual compression or proximal control with vessel loops or clamps. Smaller arterial injuries are often amenable to primary repair, whereas bigger injuries may possibly require grafting [11, 12]. If nephrectomy is required, then working status of the contralateral kidney must be confirmed.

14.3.3 Zone III Retroperitoneal Injuries

The indications for exploring blunt Zone III injuries are expanding and pulsatile hematomas and absent distal pulsations. Surgical exploration and preperitoneal packing and pelvic angiography and angioembolization should be considered for hematomas or active extravasation of contrast in Zone III from blunt injury depending upon the hemodynamic status of the patient. During surgical exploration, the iliac artery is exposed by taking out the entire small bowel from the peritoneal cavity. Following this the vessel is controlled both proximally and distally. After this the meticulous dissection of the ureter, which crosses at bifurcation of iliac vessels of that side, is done before attempting any repair. For minor injuries of the vessel, primary repair is recommended, while larger injuries can be resected with end-to-end repair, and/or grafting (PTFE or saphenous vein interposition) may be utilized. Very often injuries to the iliac arteries may be associated with hollow viscus injuries which also need addressing. In case the patient is unstable, consideration should be given to temporary intravascular shunts TIVS as damage control measure to maintain the flow of blood to the lower extremity and prevent the development of ischemic insult to the lower extremity. Ligation of the iliac veins can be considered for large injuries or in unstable patients as the ligation of the common or external iliac vein is well tolerated with few adverse effects [13].

With advent of endovascular treatment, various definitive and temporary options are available. Temporary balloon occlusion may be a time-buying procedure till the patient is shifted to the operation room and bleeding point is delineated. Another option is coil or Gelfoam angiographic embolization of the internal iliac artery or its branches.

References

1. Reinberg O, Yazbeck S. Major perineal trauma in children. J Pediatr Surg. 1989;24:982–4.
2. Ameh EA. Anorectal injuries in children. Pediatr Surg Int. 2000;16:388–91.
3. Nakayama DN. Abdominal and genitourinary trauma. In: O'Neil JA, Grosfeld JL, Fonkalsrud EW, Coran AG, Caldamone AA, editors. Principles of pediatric surgery. 2nd ed. Maryland Heights, MO: Mosby; 2004. p. 159–75.

4. Snyder CL. Abdominal and genitourinary trauma. In: Ashcraft KW, Murphy JP, Sharp RJ, et al., editors. Pediatric surgery. Philadelphia: Saunders; 2000. p. 204.

5. Mihos P, Potaris K, Gakidis J, et al. Traumatic rupture of the diaphragm: experience with 65 patients. Injury. 2003;34:169–72.

6. Coimbra R, Yang J, Hoyt DB. Injuries of the abdominal aorta and inferior vena cava in association with thoracolumbar fractures: a lethal combination. J Trauma. 1996;41:533–5.

7. Asensio JA, Petrone P, Garcia-Nunez L, et al. Superior mesenteric venous injuries: to ligate or to repair remains the question. J Trauma. 2007;62:668–75.

8. Hansen CJ, Bernadas C, West MA, et al. Abdominal vena caval injuries: outcomes remain dismal. Surgery. 2000;128:572–8.

9. Coimbra R, Filho AR, Nesser RA, et al. Outcome from traumatic injury of the portal and superior mesenteric veins. Vasc Endovasc Surg. 2004;38:249–55.

10. Arvieu C, Cardin N, Chiche L, Bachellier P, Falcon D, Letoublon C, et al. Damage control laparotomy for haemorrhagic abdominal trauma. A retrospective multicentric study about 109 cases. Ann Chir. 2003;128(3):150–8.

11. Asensio JA, Petrone P, Roldan G, et al. Analysis of 185 iliac vessel injuries: risk factors and predictors of outcome. Arch Surg. 2003;138:1187–93. discussion 1193–4.

12. Ball CG, Feliciano DV. Damage control techniques for common and external iliac artery injuries: have temporary intravascular shunts replaced the need for ligation? J Trauma. 2010;68:1117–20.

13. DuBose J, Inaba K, Barmparas G, et al. Bilateral internal iliac artery ligation as a damage control approach in massive retroperitoneal bleeding after pelvic fracture. J Trauma. 2010;69:1507–14.